PSYCHOPHA͟ ͟GY:
CLINICIAN'S ͟ ͟ ͟

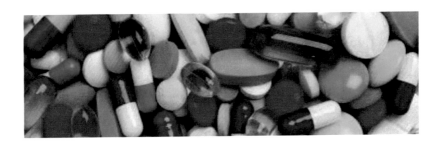

Author:
James Viola, PharmD, BCPP
Clinical Pharmacist, Mental Health-Veterans Administration
Sterile Compounding Pharmacist, Per Diem-Mayo Clinic
Adjunct Clinical Assistant Professor of Pharmacy
University of Florida
Board Certified Psychiatric Pharmacist

Contributing Author/Editor:
Jennifer Warzynski, PharmD, BCPS
Psychiatric Pharmacy Resident-Veterans Administration
Board Certified Pharmacotherapy Specialist

Published by PINK LABEL DESIGNS, LLC, St. Augustine, FL © 2017

Table of Contents

The majority of dosing throughout this book is for adult dosing.
Reduced dosing is often necessary for geriatric and pediatric patients.

Pharmacokinetics and Bioequivalence

This section includes:
- A general overview of active metabolites and enantiomers
- A general overview of bioequivalence
- A general overview of pharmacokinetics

Manufacturers may attempt to market an active metabolite, isomer or new salt form of the original drug as that particular drug patent approaches expiration. This is done to retain market share and continue company earnings. These newer versions are often known as "purified," "me too," "follow-on," or "patent extender" drugs. The new drugs name will be prefixed with "es," "ar," "lev" or "dextro." In some cases, the new formulations may have a better "cleaner" drug interaction or side effect profile compared to original version. The isomers look identical and are known as enantiomers which are mirror images (i.e. left & right shoe).[1-3]

Active Metabolites: Often begin with **"Des"**

INITIAL DRUG	ACTIVE METABOLITE
Imipramine (Tofranil®)	**Des**ipramine (Norpramin®)
Loratadine (Claritin®)	**Des**loratadine (Clarinex®)
Venlafaxine (Effexor®)	**Des**venlafaxine (Pristiq™)
Active Metabolites As Other Medications Without DES Prefix	
Amitriptyline (Elavil®)	Nortriptyline (Pamelor®)
Loxapine (Loxitane®)	Amoxapine (Asendin®)
Risperidone (Risperdal®)	Paliperidone (Invega®)

Enantiomers: Right: D- prefix (Dextro) & R (Ar)- prefix (Rectus)

INITIAL DRUG	ENANTIOMER
Amphetamine (Benzedrine™)	Dextroamphetamine (Dexedrine®)
Chlorpheniramine (Chlor-Trimeton®)	Dexchlorpheniramine (Polaramine®)
Fenfluramine (Pondimin®)	Dexfenfluramine (Redux®)
Lansoprazole (Prevacid®)	Dexlansoprazole (Dexilant® or Kapidex™)
Methylphenidate (Ritalin®)	Dexmethylphenidate (Focalin®)
Modafinil (Provigil®)	Armodafinil (Nuvigil®)
Formoterol (Foradil®)	Arformoterol (Brovana®)

INITIAL DRUG	ENANTIOMER
Albuterol (Ventolin®)	Levalbuterol (Xopenex®)
Bupivacaine (Marcaine®)	Levobupivacaine (Chirocaine®)
Cetirizine (Zyrtec®)	Levocetirizine (Xyzal®)
Milnacipran (Savella®)	Levomilnacipran (Fetzima®)
Ofloxacin (Floxin™)	Levofloxacin (Levaquin®)
Citalopram (Celexa®)	Escitalopram (Lexapro®)
Omeprazole (Prilosec®)	Esomeprazole (Nexium®)
Zopiclone (Imovane®)	Eszopiclone (Lunesta®)

Bioequivalence:

Bioequivalence means the active ingredient of two products has the same rate of absorption (C_{max}) and extent of absorption (AUC). The average values for C_{max} and AUC and degree of variability are calculated as these parameters are determined for a group of persons taking the test drug and another group of persons taking the reference drug. The limit of C_{max} and AUC ratios must be 80%. Being the data is log-transformed the upper limit of the ratio must be 125% (Reciprocal of lower limit=1/80%).

Bioequivalence Range: 80-125%

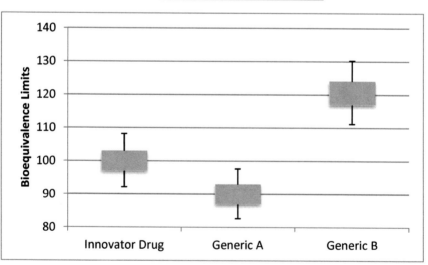

Generic A is bioequivalent to the innovator drug- the error bars overlap, and falls within 80-125%.

Generic B is NOT equivalent to the innovator drug- the error bars do not overlap with innovator drug, and falls out of 80-125% range.

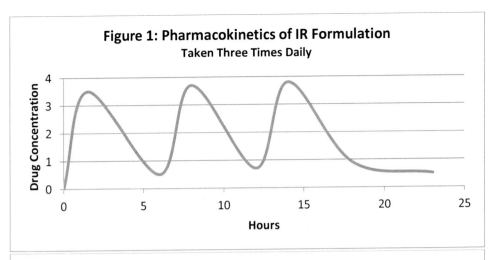

Figure 1: Pharmacokinetics of IR Formulation
Taken Three Times Daily

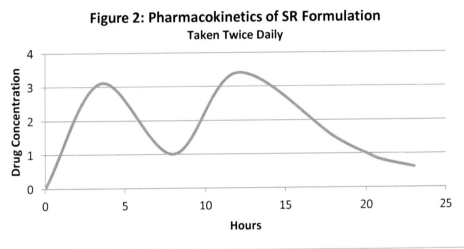

Figure 2: Pharmacokinetics of SR Formulation
Taken Twice Daily

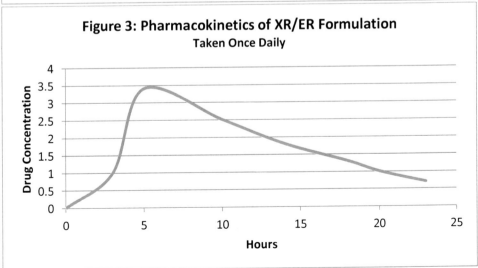

Figure 3: Pharmacokinetics of XR/ER Formulation
Taken Once Daily

Anxiolytics & Hypnotics
(Benzodiazepines, "Z" drugs, Miscellaneous)

There are many different anxiety disorders: Generalized Anxiety Disorder (GAD), Obsessive-Compulsive Disorder (OCD), Panic Disorder (PD), Post-Traumatic Disorder (PTSD) and Social Anxiety Disorder (SAD). First line treatment for these conditions are SSRI & SNRI agents.

This section includes:
- A general overview of benzodiazepines, alternative anxiolytics and hypnotic medications
- Classes of medication charts
- Dose form, route and dosage range table
- Pharmacokinetics table
- FDA approved uses

Benzodiazepine Metabolism Pathway

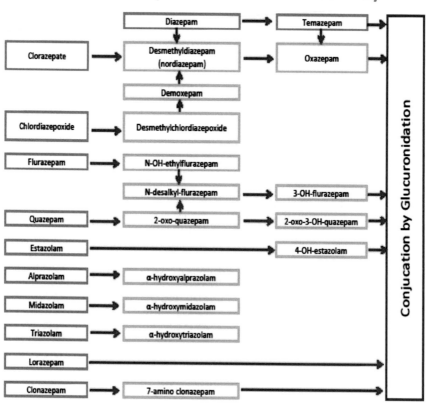

Table 1 describes dosage form, route of administration, and usual daily dose of various anxiolytics and hypnotics:

Generic Name	Brand Name	Dosage Form*	Route	Dose Range^
Benzodiazepines				
Alprazolam	Xanax®/XR®	ERT, L ODT, T	PO	0.25-10 mg/day ÷
Chlordiazepoxide	Librium®	C	PO	5-25 mg TID-QID; EtOH w/d: 50-100 mg Q4-6 hours
Clobazam	Onfi®	T, L	PO	5-20 mg BID
Clonazepam	Klonopin®/ Wafers®	ODT, T	PO	0.25-20 mg/day ÷
Clorazepate	Tranxene SD®/T-Tab®	T	PO	7.5-90 mg/day ÷
Diazepam	Diastat®/ Valium®	L, R, SI, T	PO/IM/ IV/Rectal	2-40 mg/day ÷
Estazolam	ProSom™	T	PO	0.5-2 mg HS
Flurazepam	Dalmane®	C	PO	15-30 mg HS
Lorazepam	Ativan®	L, SI, T	PO/IM/IV	1-10 mg/day ÷
Midazolam	Versed®	L, SI	PO/IM/IV	1-20 mg/day
Oxazepam	Serax®	C	PO	10-30 mg TID-QID
Quazepam	Doral®	T	PO	7.5-15 HS
Temazepam	Restoril™	C	PO	7.5-30 mg HS
Triazolam	Halcion®	T	PO	0.125-0.5 mg HS
"Z" Drugs				
Eszopiclone	Lunesta®	T	PO	1-3 mg HS
Zaleplon	Sonata®	C	PO	5-20 mg HS
Zolpidem	Ambien®/CR® Edluar® Intermezzo® Zolpimist®	ERT, OS, SL, T	PO/SL	IR/SL/Spray: 5-10 mg HS ER:6.25-12.5 mg HS SL (Intermezzo): 1.75-3.5 mg HS
Miscellaneous				
Belsomra	Suvorexant®	T	PO	5-20 mg HS
Buspirone	BuSpar®	T	PO	7.5-30 mg BID
Hydroxyzine	Atarax®; Vistaril®	C, L, T	PO	50-100 mg QID
Ramelteon	Rozerem®	T	PO	8 mg HS

*C: Capsule, L: Liquid for oral use, ERT: Extended-Release Tablet, ODT: Orally Disintegrating Tablet, OS: oral spray; R: Rectal Gel, SI: Solution/suspension for injection, T: Tablet, SL: Sublingual Tablets; ^÷: Divided, EtOH: Alcohol.

Table 2 describes various pharmacokinetic profiles of anxiolytics/hypnotics:

Drug	MOA	$T_{1/2}$ (Hours)*	Metabolism^	Enzyme Inhibited
Benzodiazepines				
Alprazolam [H]	BZD	IR:11.2; ER: 10.7-15.8	CYP 3A4	N/A
Chlordiaz-epoxide [H, R]	BZD	14-100	Oxidation	N/A
Clobazam [H]	BZD	36-42; *71-82*	CYPs 3A4 & 2C19 & 2B6	Inhibits CYP2D6 Weak Inducer CYP3A4
Clonazepam [H, R]	BZD	30-40	CYP3A4	N/A
Clorazepate [H]	BZD	30-200	Hydroxylation; Glucuronidation	N/A
Diazepam [H, R]	BZD	30-100	CYPs 3A4 & 2C19	N/A
Estazolam [H, R]	BZD	10-24	CYP 3A	N/A
Flurazepam [H, R]	BZD	30-100	Oxidation	N/A
Lorazepam [R]	BZD	12	Glucuronidation	N/A
Midazolam [H, R]	BZD	1.8-6.4	Hydroxylation; CYP 3A4	N/A
Oxazepam	BZD	5-15	Glucuronidation	N/A
Quazepam [H, R]	BZD	39-73	CYP3A4; partial CYPs 2C9/19	N/A
Temazepam	BZD	8-15	Glucuronidation	N/A
Triazolam [H]	BZD	1.5-5.5	CYP3A4	N/A
"Z" Drugs				
Eszopiclone [H]	"Z"	6	CYP 3A4 & 2E1	N/A
Zaleplon [H]	"Z"	1	CYP 3A4	N/A
Zolpidem [H]	"Z"	2.5	CYP 3A4	N/A
Miscellaneous				
Belsomra [H]	O Antag	12	CYP 3A & 2C19	Potential Inhibition of CYP 3A & P-gp
Buspirone [H, R]	5HT1 Partial Agonist	2-3	CYP 3A4	N/A
Hydroxyzine [H, R]	H_1 Antag	14-25	CYP P450	Weak CYP2D6 Inhibition
Ramelteon [H]	M1/2 Agonist	1-2.6	CYP 1A2	N/A

[H] caution advised in hepatic impairment [R] caution advised in renal impairment
*After Oral Administration. Italicized represents $T_{1/2}$ of active metabolite. ^CYP: Cytochrome. BZD: benzodiazepine, H_1 Antag: antihistamine, "Z": non-benzodiazepine hypnotic, O Antag: orexin antagonist, M1 & M2: melatonin 1 & melatonin 2 agonist

Clinical Pearls

- ALL benzodiazepines carry Black Box Warning (BBW) to avoid coadministration with other CNS depressants, especially opioids, unless no other alternatives are available. [42]
- ALL benzodiazepines carry Black Box Warning (BBW) with coadministration with respiratory depression--avoid in pulmonary disease if possible due to increased risk of respiratory depression.
- Physiologic dependence can occur with therapeutic doses as few as 3-6 weeks and with a very high prevalence within 4 months to 1 year of continued use. Risk of dependence increases with higher daily dosages and long-term treatment. For those who may dependent and require drug discontinuation the benzodiazepine should be gradually tapered.
- Withdrawal symptoms are commonly seen if the benzodiazepine (BZD) is stopped abruptly or withdrawn too quickly. They are more likely to occur and of greater intensity with BZDs that have a short duration of action. During withdrawal, the greatest risk of seizure is during the first 24-72 hours and are greater risk for seizure if on other drugs that lower the seizure threshold. [1]
- The federal Omnibus Budget Reconciliation Act (OBRA) regulates the use of sedatives/hypnotics in long-term care facility (LTCF) residents. Facility should attempt quarterly tapers unless clinically contraindicated. [47]
- Smoking can enhance the metabolism of some benzodiazepines.
- Beers Criteria from American Geriatrics Society strongly recommend the BZD class should not be used to treat insomnia, agitation or delirium in patients over 65 years old.[50]
- Should be avoided in all patients with cognitive impairment, dementia and history of falls or fractures.
- Reduced dosing in geriatrics is recommended— (If BZD required in geriatric or hepatically impaired patient, lorazepam, oxazepam, and temazepam are preferred).

> **"Outside The Liver"**
> Lorazepam
> Oxazepam
> Temazepam

The benzodiazepines (BZDs) have a wide variety of indications (insomnia, anxiety disorders, seizure disorders, anesthesia and sedation, skeletal muscle relaxation and alcohol withdrawal.) The individual drugs can be distinguished by their various pharmacokinetic profiles (long-acting, medium-acting and short-acting,) onset of action (rapid, intermediate or slow) and metabolic pathways (CYP P450 versus conjugation/glucuronidation).

Table 3 describes various FDA approved indications for drugs used for anxiolytics and hypnotics:

	GAD	OCD	PD	Insomnia	Seizure Disorder	EtOH W/D	Misc.
Benzodiazepines							
Alprazolam	X		X				
Chlordiaz-epoxide	X					X	
Clobazam					X		*Adjunctive treatment of Lennox-Gastaut syndrome*
Clonazepam			X		X		
Clorazepate	X				*X*	X	*Adjunctive treatment of partial seizures*
Diazepam	X				X		Multiple*
Estazolam				X			
Flurazepam				X			
Lorazepam	X			X	X		Multiple*
Midazolam							Multiple*
Oxazepam	X					X	
Quazepam				X			
Temazepam				X			
Triazolam				X			
"Z" Drugs							
Eszopiclone				X			
Zaleplon				X			
Zolpidem				X			
Miscellaneous							
Belsomra				X			
Buspirone	X						
Hydroxyzine	X						
Ramelteon				X			
GAD: Generalized Anxiety Disorder, OCD: Obsessive Compulsive Disorder, PD: Panic Disorder, EtOH W/D: Alcohol Withdrawal). *See Clinical Pearls							

Benzodiazepines (BZDs) [48-49]

MOA: BZDs bind nonspecifically to BZD_1 & BZD_2 which ultimately enhance GABA. GABA is an inhibitory neurotransmitter that exerts its effects at specific receptor subtypes ($GABA_A$ & $GABA_B$.) $GABA_A$ is primarily involved in actions of anxiolytics and sedatives. There are specific receptors located in the CNS and tissue. BZD_1 is located in the cerebellum & cerebral cortex (thought to mediate sleep,) BZD_2 is in the cerebral cortex & spinal cord (affect muscle relaxation) and BZD_3 is in the peripheral tissues.

Adverse Effects: confusion, dizziness, drowsiness, falls, fatigue, impaired cognition, memory impairment and xerostomia are all common side effects.

Contraindications: benzodiazepine hypersensitivity or known allergy to any component of formulation. Many BZDs are contraindicated in close-angle glaucoma. Some are contraindicated in myasthenia gravis and sleep apnea. Relative contraindication with history of substance abuse.

Benzodiazepine Approximate Dose Equivalencies [43]

Drug	Onset	Duration	Approximate Equivalency
Alprazolam	Rapid	Short	0.5 mg
Chlordiazepoxide	Intermediate	Long	12.5 mg
Clobazam	Slow	Long	N/A
Clonazepam	Rapid	Intermediate	0.25-0.5 mg
Clorazepate	Intermediate	Long	7.5 mg
Diazepam	Rapid	Long	5 mg
Estazolam	Intermediate	Intermediate	0.5 mg
Flurazepam	Rapid	Long	7.5 mg
Lorazepam	Rapid	Intermediate	1 mg
Midazolam	Rapid	Short	N/A
Oxazepam	Slow	Intermediate	15 mg
Quazepam	Intermediate	Long	5 mg
Temazepam	Intermediate	Intermediate	7.5 mg
Triazolam	Rapid	Short	0.125 mg

Alprazolam (Xanax®/XR®) [2-5]

Available: 0.25, 0.5, 1, 2 mg tablets; 0.25, 0.5, 1, 2 mg oral disintegrating tablets (ODT); 0.5, 1, 2, 3 mg extended release tablets; 1 mg/1 mL oral solution

Dose: **GAD:** 0.25-0.5 mg TID; may increase dose at intervals of 3-4 days to max of 4 mg/day. **PD:** 0.5 mg TID; may increase dose at intervals of 3-4 days to a max of 10 mg/day. **ER tablet:** 0.5-1 mg QAM; may increase dose at intervals of 3-4 days; to a max of 10 mg/day.

Renal: No adjustment.

Hepatic: Consider initial *dose reduction*; titrate as needed/tolerated

- Taper to discontinuation; manufacturer suggest daily dose be decreased by no more than 0.5 mg every 3 days. Some patients require a more gradual and individualized taper.
- **Caution with CYP 3A4 inhibitors**; contraindicated with Ketoconazole & Itraconazole due to Potent CYP 3A4 inhibition.
- Contraindicated in closed-angle glaucoma

Chlordiazepoxide (Librium®) [6]

Available: 5, 10, 25 mg capsules

Dose: **Anxiety:** 5-10 mg TID-QID for mild/moderate anxiety and 20-25 mg TID-QID for severe anxiety with max Dose of 100 mg/day. **EtOH withdrawal:** 50-100 mg followed by repeated dose every 4-6 hours until agitation controlled with max Dose of 300 mg/day.

Renal: *CrCl < 10 mL/min:* reduce by 50%

Hepatic: Use with *caution*; repeated dosing results in accumulation

Clobazam (Onfi®) [7]

Available: 10, 20 mg tablets; 2.5 mg/mL liquid solution

Dose: **Lennox-Gastaut (LGS) adjunctive treatment:** *Weight > 30kg*: 5 mg BID X 6 days → 10 mg BID X 7 days → 20 mg BID. *Weight < 30kg*: 5 mg Qdaily x 6 days → 5 mg BID x 7 days → 10 mg BID.

Renal: No adjustment

Hepatic: *>30kg with mild/moderate impairment (Child-Pugh 5-9):* 5 mg daily for 6 days → 5 mg BID x 7 days → 10 mg BID x 7 days. Day 21-may increase to 10 mg BID. *≤30kg: with mild/moderate impairment (Child-Pugh 5-9):* 5 mg daily for 6 days → 5 mg BID x 7 days. Day 21-may increase to 10 mg BID.

- Doses above 5 mg/day must be divided in two doses
- **Dose adjustments for geriatric patients, mild/moderate hepatic impairment and know CYP2C19 poor metabolizers**
- Reduce by 5-10 mg/day on a weekly basis to discontinue[3]

Clonazepam (Klonopin®/Wafers®) [8-9]

Available: 0.125, 0.25, 0.5, 1 and 2 mg oral disintegrating tablets (ODT); 0.5, 1 and 2 mg tablets

Dose: **PD:** 0.25 mg BID; may increase to 1 mg/day after 3 days. May increase gradually as needed by 0.125-0.25mg BID Q3 days. Max Dose of 4 mg/day.
Seizure Disorder: *Weight > 30 kg*: 0.5 mg TID; may increase by 0.5-1 mg every 3 days until seizures controlled. Max Dose of 20 mg/day. *Weight < 30kg*: 0.01-0.03 mg/kg/day (divided 3 equal doses) and may increase by 0.25-0.5 mg every 3rd day. Max Dose of 0.05 mg/kg/day (divided BID-TID).

Renal: *Modify* depending upon clinical response & degree of impairment
Hepatic: *Modify* depending upon clinical response & degree of impairment

- Effective in prophylaxis of the following seizures: absence, petit mal variant (Lennox-Gastaut Syndrome,) akinetic and myoclonic & nocturnal myoclonus. It is not effective for generalized tonic-clonic seizures.
- Contraindicated in closed-angle glaucoma and severe hepatic disease

Clorazepate (Tranxene SD®/T-Tab®) [10]

Available: 3.75, 7.5, 15mg tablets

Dose: **EtOH withdrawal:** Day 1: 30 mg followed by 30-60 mg in divided doses, Day 2: 45-90 mg in divided doses, Day 3: 22.5-45 mg in divided doses, Day 4: 15-30 mg in divided doses and gradually reduce to 7.5-15 mg to taper off. Max dose of 90 mg/day. **Anxiety:** 15 mg HS; usual dose 30 mg/day in divided doses. Max dose of 60 mg/day. **Partial seizures:** 7.5 mg BID-TID may increase by 7.5 mg per week. Max dose of 90 mg/day in adults and 60 mg/day in children 9-12 years old.

Renal: No adjustment
Hepatic: Dosing *may need to be altered* to compensate for impaired hepatic metabolism

- Contraindicated in closed-angle glaucoma

Diazepam (Diastat®; Valium®) [11-14]

Available: 2, 5, 10 mg tablets; 5 mg/mL intensol & 5 mg/5 mL & oral solutions; 5 mg/mL solution for injection; 2.5, 10, 20 mg rectal gel

Dose: **Anxiety:** *PO:* 2-10 mg BID-QID depending upon severity of symptoms. Max Dose commonly implied limit is 40 mg/day. *IM/IV:* 2-5mg for moderate anxiety and 5-10 mg for severe anxiety; may repeat in 3-4 hours. **Acute EtOH withdrawal:** 10 mg IV initially; followed by 5-10 mg every 3-4 hours as needed. Some patients require massive doses during acute phase. **Muscle spasm:** *PO:* 2-10 mg TID-QID. *IV/IM:* 5-10 mg initially; repeat every 3-4 hours as needed. **Status Epilepticus:** 5-10 mg IV, repeated at 10-15 minute intervals to a max dose of 30 mg. May repeat in 2-4 hours if needed.

Renal: *Modify* depending upon clinical response & degree of impairment
Hepatic: *Modify* depending upon clinical response & degree of impairment

- Additionally approved for amnesia induction, muscle spasm, sedation induction, tetanus
- Contraindicated in closed-angle glaucoma, severe hepatic disease, myasthenia gravis, infants/neonates, respiratory insufficiency and sleep apnea

Estazolam (ProSom™) [15]
Available: 1, 2mg tablets
Dose: 1 mg HS; may increase to 2mg HS
Renal: *CrCl < 10 ml/min:* may require dose reduction up to 50%.
Hepatic: *Modify* depending upon clinical response & degree of impairment.

Flurazepam (Dalmane®) [16-17]
Available: 15, 30 mg capsules
Dose: 15 mg HS; may increase to 30 mg HS.
Renal: *CrCl 10-80 mL/min:* initiate with lowest recommended dose & adjust per clinical response. *CrCl < 10 mL/min:* monitor closely-CNS effect may increase due to decreased elimination.
Hepatic: *Modify* depending upon clinical response & degree of impairment

Lorazepam (Ativan®) [18-20]
Available: 2 mg/ml intensol oral solution; 0.5, 1, 2 mg tablets; 2 mg/mL & 4 mg/mL solution for injection
Dose: **Anxiety:** *PO:* 1 mg BID-TID; increase gradually as needed/tolerated. Usual dose is 2-6 mg/day. Max Dose of 10 mg/day. **Insomnia:** *PO:* 2-4 mg QHS as needed. Max Dose of 4 mg/day. **Status Epilepticus:** *IV:* 4 mg slowly (2 mg/min) may be followed by additional 4 mg after 10-15 minutes if needed.
Renal: *Modify* depending upon clinical response & degree of impairment
Hepatic: No adjustment
- Additionally approved for amnesia induction, sedation induction and seizures (status epilepticus)
- Lorazepam & midazolam are the most commonly used agents in which they are administered parenterally (IM/IV) in hospital settings (ICU/ER)
- Contraindicated in benzyl alcohol hypersensitivity (some injectable forms,) closed-angle glaucoma, intra-arterial admin and sleep apnea.

Midazolam (Versed®) [21]
Available: 2 mg/mL oral solution; 1 mg/mL & 5 mg/mL solution for injection
Dose: *PO:* 0.25-0.5 mg/kg as single dose 30-45 minutes prior to procedure. Max Dose of 20 mg. *IV:* 1-5 mg over 2-minute period immediately prior to procedure. *IM:* 0.07-0.08 mg/kg (~5 mg for average healthy adult) 30-60 minutes prior to surgery.
Renal: *Modify* depending upon clinical response & degree of impairment

Hepatic: *Modify* depending upon clinical response & degree of impairment
- Additionally approved for IM/IV preoperative sedation/anxiolysis/amnesia; IV sedation/anxiolysis/amnesia during diagnostic, therapeutic or endoscopic procedures; IV for general anesthesia prior to other anesthetic agents; continuous IV infusion for sedation of intubated & mechanically ventilated patients.
- High incidence of partial/complete impairment of recall for several hours.
- Midazolam and lorazepam are the most commonly used agents in which they are administered parenterally (IM/IV) in hospital settings (ICU/ER)
- Clinical experience has shown midazolam to be **3 to 4 times** as potent per mg as diazepam.
- Contraindicated in closed-angle glaucoma and epidural admin.

Oxazepam (Serax®) [22]
Available: 10, 15, 30 mg capsules
Dose: **GAD:** 10-15 mg TID-QID for mild/moderate anxiety & 15-30 mg TID-QID for severe anxiety. Max Dose of 120 mg/day. **EtOH withdrawal:** 15-30 mg TID-QID.
Renal: No adjustment
Hepatic: No adjustment

Quazepam (Doral®) [23]
Available: 7.5, 15 mg tablets
Dose: 7.5-15 mg HS.
Renal: *Modify* depending upon clinical response & degree of impairment.
Hepatic: *Modify* depending upon clinical response & degree of impairment.
- Contraindicated in closed-angle glaucoma and sleep apnea.

Temazepam (Restoril™) [24]
Available: 7.5, 15, 22.5, 30 mg capsules
Dose: 15 mg HS (30 minutes before bed) may increase to 30 mg HS.
Renal: No adjustment.
Hepatic: No adjustment.

Triazolam (Halcion®) [25]
Available: 0.125, 0.25 mg tablets
Dose: 0.125-0.25 mg HS with Max Dose of 0.5 mg HS.
Renal: No adjustment.
Hepatic: Initial dose of 0.125 mg in impairment.
- Many reports of retrograde amnesia
- Indicated for short-term use (generally 7-10 days). Use for more than 2-3 weeks requires re-evaluation of patient.

"Z" Medications

MOA: Modulates GABA-A subunit (aka GABA-BZ or omega receptor) with high affinity for BZ1 α1/ α5 subunits (hence lack of myorelaxant & anticonvulsant effects) and helps to preserve deep sleep (stages 3 & 4).

Adverse Effects: most of the adverse effects tend to be dose-related & CNS-related. Dizziness, lightheadedness, headache, memory impairment, amnesia, anterograde amnesia, complex sleep-related behaviors (somnambulism, sleep-driving, sleep shopping, making phone calls, having sex, preparing/eating food while not fully awake, generally with amnesia of event have occurred.)

Contraindications: Hypersensitivity to particular product

Eszopiclone (Lunesta®) [26]

Available: 1, 2, 3 mg tablets

Dose: 1 mg QHS may increase to 2-3 mg QHS. Max Dose of 3 mg QHS.

Renal: No adjustment

Hepatic: *Severe impairment* should receive initial dose of 1mg HS and should not receive more than 2 mg at bedtime.

- Must have at least 7-8 hours remaining before planned time of awakening
- **Reduce dose in CYP 3A4 Inhibitors (no more than 2 mg QHS)**
- Often associated with unpleasant (metallic) taste
- Avoid with/immediately after a meal--slower absorption/reduced effect

Zaleplon (Sonata®) [27]

Available: 5, 10 mg capsules

Dose: 10 mg QHS; may increase to 20 mg HS if no benefit from 10 mg dose.

Renal: No adjustment.

Hepatic: Initial dose of 5 mg HS for *mild/moderate impairment*. Not recommended in *severe impairment*.

- Must be provided with at least 4 or more hours of sleep
- Effects may be reduced if taken with/immediately after high-fat meal

Zolpidem (Ambien®/CR®; Edluar®; Intermezzo®; Zolpimist®) [28-33]

Available: 5, 10 mg tablets; 6.25 mg, 12.5 mg extended-release tablets; 5 mg/actuation lingual spray; 1.75, 3.5, 5, 10 mg sublingual tablets

Dose: **PO/SL:** Women- 5 mg HS initially; Men- 5-10 mg HS. **Oral Spray:** Women- 1 spray (5 mg) HS; Men- 1-2 sprays (5-10 mg HS). **ER:** Women- 6.25 mg HS initially; Men- 6.25-12.5 mg HS. Max Dose: IR/SL/Spray is 10 mg/day. ER is 12.5 mg/day. At least 7-8 hours required before next morning awakening.

SL-Intermezzo®: Middle-of-the-night awakening with at least 4 hours before awakening: Women-1.75 mg HS & Men 3.5 mg HS. Max Dose is 3.5 mg HS.

Renal: No adjustment

Hepatic: Due to hepatic clearance, *lower doses are recommended. 5 mg/day for IR (Ambien®)/Lingual Spray (Zolpimist®)/SL (Edluar®), 6.25mg/day for ER (Ambien CR®), 1.75 mg/day for SL (Intermezzo®)*

- Clearance is lower in women--plasma levels may be elevated next morning enough to impair activities requiring mental alertness (i.e. driving.)
- Effects may be slowed if taken with/immediately after a meal.
- Risk for next-morning impairment is higher with extended-release tablets.
- Zolpimist-After initial priming of 5 actuations, there are 60 actuations. If not used ≥ 14 days requires to be primed again with 1 spray.

Miscellaneous

Belsomra (Suvorexant®) [34]
Available: 5, 10, 15 and 20 mg tablets
Dose: 10mg HS (30 minutes before bed.) If 10 mg dose well-tolerated but not effective the dose may be increased. Max Dose: 20 mg/day.
Renal: No adjustment
Hepatic: Not recommended in *severe impairment*
MOA: Antagonism of orexin receptors (blocks binding of wake-promoting neuropeptides orexin A and orexin B to receptors OX1R and OX2R).

- CYP 3A inhibitors-initial dose of 5 mg HS and may increase to 10 mg HS
- **NOT RECOMMENDED WITH STRONG CYP 3A INHIBITORS**
- **DO NOT USE IN NARCOLEPSY**
- Should not be used with other drugs to treat insomnia
- Give at least 7 hours before planned awakening
- Give without food for faster onset
- Monitor digoxin concentrations if used concomitantly

Buspirone (BuSpar®) [35]
Available: 5, 7.5, 10, 15, 30mg tablets
Dose: 7.5 mg BID, then increase by 5 mg/day every 2-3 days. Max Dose of 60 mg/day.
Renal: *CrCl 11-70 mL/min:* modify dose by 25-50% and adjust based upon clinical response. *CrCl ≤ 10mL/min:* avoid use.
Hepatic: *Modify* dose by 25-50% based upon clinical response. *Avoid* use in severe impairment.
MOA: Partial $5HT_{1A}$ agonism and moderate affinity for D_2 receptors

- Dose adjustments may be necessary when administered with CYP 3A4 Inhibitors or Inducers
- Onset of anxiolytic effect may take between 2-6 weeks

Hydroxyzine (Atarax®; Vistaril®) [36-38]

Available: 10, 25, 50 mg tablets; 25, 50, 100 mg capsules; 10 mg/5mL oral solution; 25 mg/5mL oral suspension

Dose: 50-100 mg QID

Renal: *CrCl ≤ 50mL/min:* reduce dose by 50%

Hepatic: *Modify* depending upon clinical response & degree of impairment

MOA: H_1 antagonist with cetirizine as one active metabolite and norchlorcyclizine as another (which has chemical similarities to a trazodone metabolite-m-chlorophenylpiperazine).

- Additionally indicated for adjunct to pre & postoperative analgesia and anesthesia, antipruritic and antiemetic. Has been used off label for insomnia at 50-100 mg HS.

Ramelteon (Rozerem®) [39, 41]

Available: 8 mg tablet

Dose: 8 mg HS

Renal: No adjustment

Hepatic: *Mild/moderate impairment:* caution; severe impairment: not recommended

MOA: Potent melatonin receptor agonist, MT1 and MT2, which are believed to be involved in regulation of circadian rhythm. MT1 is suggested to regulate sleepiness and MT2 to help shift body between day and night.

- Not recommended with or after high-fat meal.

Flumazenil (Romazicon®) [40]

Available: 0.1 mg/1 mL solution for injection

Dose: Initially 0.2 mg IV; additional dose of 0.3 mg IV 30 seconds later if desired level of consciousness not achieved. Further dose of 0.5mg may be administered at 1-minute intervals up to Max Dose of 3 mg (rarely 5 mg).

Renal: No adjustment

Hepatic: No adjustment

- For reversal of benzodiazepine toxicity in suspected overdose or post procedure reversal

Off label use for anxiety and/or insomnia: [44-46, 56]

Propranolol: 10-80 mg given 1 hour prior to anxiety provoking event.

Melatonin: 0.3-10 mg HS for sleep.

Trazodone: 25-100 mg HS for sleep.

Valerian: 400-450 mg BID-TID or 400-450mg HS for sleep.

Kava Kava: 40-70 mg BID-TID or 150 mg HS for sleep. (*High potential for drug-drug interactions due to multiple CYP inhibitions and caution with hepatic disease*)

Antidepressants

The antidepressant (AD) classes have a wide array of uses. They serve in the treatment of several disorders including depression, panic/anxiety disorders, obsessive-compulsive disorder (OCD) and a variety of other conditions and various illnesses.

This section includes:
- DSM-V definition of depression
- Phases and length of AD treatment
- A general overview of antidepressants
- Antidepressant Discontinuation Syndrome (ADS)
- Classes of medication charts
- Dose form, route and dosage range table
- Pharmacokinetics table
- FDA approved uses table
- Clinical pearls

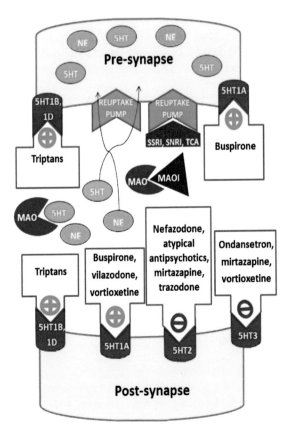

The figure to the left represents mechanism of action for various drugs often used for depression. The (+) sign represents agonist effects and (-) represents antagonist effects of drugs on various serotonin (5HT) receptors. Various selective serotonin reuptake inhibitors (SSRI), serotonin and norepinephrine reuptake inhibitors (SNRI) and tricyclic antidepressants (TCA) block the reuptake pump, which allows more 5HT and norepinephrine (NE) to stay within the synapse. Monoamine oxidases (MAO), which are responsible for degrading 5HT and NE, are inhibited by monoamine oxidase inhibitors (MAOI). This also results in increased amounts of 5HT and NE to stay within the synapse.

DIAGNOSTIC CRITERIA (DSM-5)

<u>Major Depressive Disorder (MDD)</u>

Characterized by ≥ 1 major depressive episode (no history of manic or mixed mood episodes)

- o Major depressive episode:
  - A. ≥5 of the following nearly every day ≥ 2 weeks. At least 1 of the symptoms is either depressed mood OR loss of interest of pleasure. Consider the acronym (SIGECAPS).

SIGECAPS
Suicide
Interest
Guilt
Energy
Concentration
Appetite
Psychomotor
Sleep

1. Depressed mood most of the time and most days
2. Decreased interest or pleasure in daily activities most of the time and most of days
3. Significant changes in weight (e.g. >5% change in a month), or appetite. Weight loss (not due to dieting) or weight gain or decrease/increase in appetite
4. Significant changes in sleep. Insomnia or hypersomnia
5. Psychomotor agitation or retardation (observable by others)
6. Fatigue/decrease in energy
7. Feelings of worthlessness or inappropriate guilt (may be delusional)
8. Decreased concentration or difficulty making decisions
9. Recurrent thoughts of death (not just fear of dying), suicidal ideations without a specific plan, or a suicide attempt or a specific plan for committing suicide

- B. Symptoms result in significant distress or impairment in daily function
- C. Symptoms not secondary to substance use (drug of abuse) or a general medical condition (hypothyroidism)

> *Update: DSM-IV states depression symptoms lasting less than 2 months following death of a loved one SHOULD NOT be considered/diagnosed as MDD ("bereavement exclusion"). This was removed from DSM-V.*

<u>Signs & Symptoms of Depression</u>

- Patient frequently present with depressed mood, irritability, anxiety, tearfulness and somatic complaints
- SIGECAPS
- May complain of vague somatic complaints with no identifiable medical cause (GI disturbance, headache, muscle pain)
- Prodromal symptoms (anxiety attack, panic attacks, phobias, irritability) may appear before full episode onset
- May present with poor hygiene, changes in weight, and social isolation
- No lab/imaging studies available for diagnosis conformation [1]

Phases of antidepressant treatment:

1. Acute phase (~6-12 weeks) seeking to obtain remission of symptoms.
2. Continuation phase (~4-9 months) seeking to prevent relapse of symptoms.
3. Maintenance phase (6 months-years) seek to prevent recurrence of MDD episode. [2,17]

> Response to treatment is defined as 50% reduction in depressive symptoms

Length of antidepressant treatment:
- 1st episode: 6 months – 1 year (50% chance of relapse)
- 2nd episode: 2 years (70% chance or relapse)
- 3rd episode or more: lifelong therapy (90% chance of relapse) [3,4,8,9,10]

> Primary treatment for depression is pharmacotherapy; however, ~ 40% will not respond to the 1st antidepressant and ~60% will experience at least one side effect.[2] Medication effect often takes 2-6 weeks with up to 12 weeks in various conditions. It is best to titrate "low and slow" for tolerability reasons and to minimize side effects.

Fertilizer/Antidepressant Analogy:

Plant fertilizer does not turn plants or grass green immediately. There is a delayed effect often (2-6 weeks.) The fertilizer needs to be absorbed and taken up by the roots of plant/grass. Antidepressants have a similar delayed therapeutic effect. There is an initial increase in neurotransmission (hence initial side effects such as nausea, diarrhea, etc.) while there is a gradual post synaptic receptor down-regulation (resulting in delayed antidepressant effect).

Antidepressant (AD) Effect and Mechanism of Action:

Increased neurotransmission begins after AD initiated. There is a gradual post-synaptic down-regulation which correlates with slow ongoing antidepressant response. Consider the analogy of fertilizer effect as below:

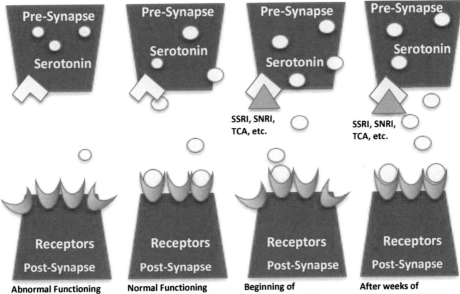

AD Initiated   4-6 WEEKS OF AD

2 WEEKS OF AD

Pre-Synapse — Serotonin

SSRI, SNRI, TCA, etc.

Receptors — Post-Synapse

Abnormal Functioning Synapse. Upregulation of post-synaptic receptors.

Normal Functioning Synapse.

Beginning of Antidepressant Therapy

After weeks of antidepressant therapy. Post-synaptic down-regulation.

19

Strategies for partial or non-response to treatment (after 4-8 weeks of adequate AD dose):
- Switching-often preferred if little/no improvement in symptoms.
- Augmentation-addition of second AD or other medication to existing AD treatment.

All ADs have potential to lower seizure threshold. ADs with highest risk (BAM): Bupropion, Amoxapine and Maprotiline [5,6]

Antidepressant Discontinuation Syndrome (ADS):

FINISH

Flu-like symptoms

Insomnia

Nausea

Imbalance

Sensory disturbance

Hyperarousal

Antidepressants are not addictive; however, they may cause serotonergic withdrawal or antidepressant discontinuation syndrome (ADS). Appears to be more common in antidepressants with short half-life ($t_{1/2}$). Paroxetine and venlafaxine are more likely to cause ADS because of its short $t_{1/2}$. Fluoxetine unlikely to result in ADS due to long $t_{1/2}$. Symptoms associated with ADS often include the "FINISH" syndrome: flu-like symptoms, insomnia, nausea, imbalance, sensory disturbance, and hyperarousal (anxiety/agitation). [7]

Table 1 describes list of tricyclic antidepressants (TCAs). The secondary amines are more specific for serotonin (5HT) than norepinephrine (NE). The tertiary amines are more specific for NE than 5HT. The red arrows ($\rightarrow$) represents metabolism to active metabolite:

Tricyclic Antidepressants (TCAs)	
Tertiary Amines (5HT > NE)	Secondary Amines (NE > 5HT)
Amitriptyline $\longrightarrow$	Nortriptyline
Clomipramine	Amoxapine
Doxepin	Maprotiline
Imipramine $\longrightarrow$	Desipramine
Trimipramine	Protriptyline

Table 2 describes list of various reuptake inhibitors, which include selective serotonin reuptake inhibitors (SSRIs) and serotonin norepinephrine reuptake inhibitors (SNRIs). The red arrows ($\rightarrow$) represent metabolism to active metabolite, and blue arrows ($\rightarrow$) represent enantiomer.

Selective Serotonin Reuptake Inhibitors (SSRIs)	Serotonin Norepinephrine Reuptake Inhibitors (SNRIs)
Citalopram	Levomilnacipran
Escitalopram	Milnacipran
Fluoxetine	Venlafaxine
Fluvoxamine	Desvenlafaxine
Paroxetine	Duloxetine
Sertraline	

Table 3 describes miscellaneous drugs and its mechanism of action.

Alpha 2 antagonist + 5HT2 & 5HT3 antagonism
Mirtazapine
Dopamine + Norepinephrine Reuptake Inhibitor (DNRI)
Bupropion
Serotonin 2 antagonist (5HT2 Antagonist)
Nefazodone
Trazodone
SSRI + 5HT1A partial agonist
Vilazodone
SSRI + 5HT1A Partial Agonist + 5HT3 Antagonist
Vortioxetine
Monoamine Oxidase Inhibitors (MAOIs)
Isocarboxazid
Phenelzine
Selegiline
Tranylcypromine

Table 4 describes various dosage forms, routes of administration, and usual daily dose range for Tricyclic Antidepressants:

Generic Name	Brand Name	Dosage Form*	Route	Dose Range
Tertiary Amines (5HT > NE)				
Amitriptyline	Elavil®	T	PO	25-300mg
Clomipramine	Anafranil®	C	PO	25-250mg
Doxepin	Silenor® Sinequan®	C, L, T	PO	3-300mg
Imipramine	Tofranil® /PM®	T, C	PO	25-300mg
Trimipramine	Surmontil®	C	PO	50-300mg
Secondary Amines (NE > 5HT)				
Amoxapine	Asendin®	T	PO	50-600mg
Desipramine	Norpramin®	T	PO	25-300mg
Maprotiline	Ludiomil®	T	PO	25-225mg
Nortriptyline	Aventyl® Pamelor®	C, L	PO	10-150mg
Protriptyline	Vivactil®	T	PO	15-60mg

C: Capsule, L: Liquid for oral use, DRC: Delayed Release Capsule, ERC: Extended-Release Capsule, ERT: Extended-Release Tablet, ODT: Orally Disintegrating Tablet, T: Tablet, SL: Sublingual Tablets, TP: Transdermal Patch.

Table 5 describes various dosage forms, routes of administration, and usual daily dose range for various reuptake inhibitors:

Generic Name	Brand Name	Dosage Form*	Route	Dose Range
Selective Serotonin Reuptake Inhibitors (SSRIs)				
Citalopram	Celexa®	T, L	PO	10-40mg
Escitalopram	Lexapro®	T, L	PO	5-20mg
Fluoxetine	Prozac®/Weekly® Sarafem® Selfemra®	C, T, L, DRC	PO	10-80mg
Fluvoxamine	Luvox® /CR®	C, ERC	PO	50-300mg
Paroxetine	Brisdelle® Paxil®/CR® Pexeva®	C, T, L, ERT	PO	10-60mg CR:12.5-75 mg
Sertraline	Zoloft®	T, L	PO	25-200mg
Serotonin Norepinephrine Reuptake Inhibitors (SNRIs)				
Desvenlafaxine	Khedezla® Pristiq®	ERT	PO	50-400mg
Duloxetine	Cymbalta® Irenka®	DRC	PO	20-120mg
Levomilnacipran	Fetzima®	ERC	PO	20-120mg
Milnacipran	Savella®	T	PO	12.5-200mg
Venlafaxine	Effexor® /XR®	C, T, ERC, ERT	PO	IR:37.5-375mg XR:37.5-225mg

*C: Capsule, L: Liquid for oral use, DRC: Delayed Release Capsule, ERC: Extended-Release Capsule, ERT: Extended-Release Tablet, T: Tablet.

Table 6 describes various dosage forms, routes of administration, and usual daily dose range for miscellaneous drugs often used for depression:

Generic Name	Brand Name	Dosage Form*	Route	Dose Range
Monoamine Oxidase Inhibitor (MAOIs)				
Isocarboxazid	Marplan®	T	PO	20-60mg
Phenelzine	Nardil®	T	PO	15-90mg
Selegiline	Carbex® Eldepryl® EMSAM® Zelapar®	C, ODT, T, TP	PO, Topical	PO:1.25-10mg Patch:6-12mg
Tranylcypromine	Parnate®	T	PO	30-60mg
Dopamine + Norepinephrine Reuptake Inhibitor (DNRI)				
Bupropion	Aplenzin® Buproban® Forfivo XL® Wellbutrin®/SR®/XL® Zyban®	T, ERT	PO	Aplenzin: 174-522mg Bupropion: IR:200-450mg SR:100-400mg XL:150-450mg

Generic Name	Brand Name	Dosage Form*	Route	Dose Range
Serotonin 2 Antagonists (5HT2 Antagonists)				
Nefazodone	Serzone®	T	PO	100-600mg
Trazodone	Desyrel® Oleptro®	T, ERC	PO	25-600mg
Alpha 2 Antagonist + 5HT2 & 5HT3 Antagonist				
Mirtazapine	Remeron® / Sol-Tab®	T, ODT	PO	7.5-45mg
SSRI + 5HT1A Partial Agonist				
Vilazodone	Viibryd®	T	PO	10-40mg
SSRI + 5HT1A Partial Agonist + 5HT3 Antagonist				
Vortioxetine	Trintellix®	T	PO	5-20mg

*C: Capsule, L: Liquid for oral use, DRC: Delayed Release Capsule, ERC: Extended-Release Capsule, ERT: Extended-Release Tablet, ODT: Orally Disintegrating Tablet, T: Tablet, SL: Sublingual Tablets, TP: Transdermal Patch

Table 7 describes various pharmacokinetic profiles of tricyclic antidepressants (TCAs) including mechanism of action (MOA), half-life ($t_{1/2}$) and metabolizing/inhibited enzymes:

Drug	MOA[#]	$T_{1/2}$ (Hours)*	Metabolism^	Enzyme Inhibited
Amitriptyline [H]	TCA	10-26; *18-44*	1A2, 3A4, 2D6 (primary)	N/A
Clomipramine[H]	TCA	32; *69*	1A2, 2C19, 2D6 (primary)	N/A
Doxepin[H]	TCA	6-8; *28-52*	1A2, 2C9/19, 2D6 (primary)	N/A
Imipramine[H]	TCA	8-16; *12-27*	1A2, 2C19, 2D6 (primary) 3A4	N/A
Trimipramine[H]	TCA	20-26	2C19, 2D6, 3A4	N/A
Amoxapine[H]	TCA	6.5-8; *30*	CYP 450 (unknown)	N/A
Desipramine[H]	TCA	12-27	2C19, 2D6 (primary)	N/A
Maprotiline[H]	TCA	27-58; *60-90*	2D6	N/A
Nortriptyline[H]	TCA	18-44	2D6	N/A
Protriptyline[H]	TCA	54-198	CYP 450 (unknown)	N/A

[H] Caution advised/adjust in hepatic impairment
[#] TCA: tricyclic antidepressant. *Half-life after oral administration. *Italicized* represents $t_{1/2}$ of active metabolite. ^CYP: Cytochrome, UGT-G: UDP-glucuronosyltransferase-Glucuronidation.

Table 8 describes various pharmacokinetic profiles of selective serotonin reuptake inhibitors (SSRIs) and serotonin norepinephrine reuptake inhibitors (SNRIs) including mechanism of action (MOA), half-life ($T_{1/2}$) and metabolizing/inhibited enzymes:

Drug	MOA[#]	$T_{1/2}$ (Hours)*	Metabolism^	Enzyme Inhibited
Citalopram[R,H]	SSRI	35	3A4, 2D6, 2C19 (primary)	Weak 2D6
Escitalopram[R,H]	SSRI	27-32	3A4, 2D6, 2C19 (primary)	Weak 2D6
Fluoxetine[H]	SSRI	4-6 DAYS; *7-9 DAYS*	2C19, 2D6 (primary)	Potent 2D6, Moderate 2C19
Fluvoxamine[H]	SSRI	16	1A2, 2D6	Potent 1A2 & 2C9 Moderate 3A4 Weak 2C9
Paroxetine[R,H]	SSRI	21-24	2D6	Potent 2D6
Sertraline[H]	SSRI	26; *66-80*	2D6, 3A4, 2C19 (primary)	>150 mg/day, Moderate 2D6
Desvenlafaxine[R,H]	SNRI	10-11	3A4 (minor) UGT	N/A
Duloxetine[R,H]	SNRI	9.2-19.1 (Avg 12.5)	1A2, 2D6	Moderate 2D6
Levomilnacipran[R]	SNRI	12	3A4 (primary) 2C8, 2C19, 2D6, 2J2, P-gp	N/A
Milnacipran[R,H]	SNRI	8-10	Minimal CYP 450 (unknown)	N/A
Venlafaxine[R,H]	SNRI	5; *11*	2D6	Weak 2D6

[H] Caution advised/adjust in hepatic impairment
[R] Caution advised/adjust in renal impairment
[#]SSRI: selective serotonin reuptake inhibitor, SNRI: serotonin norepinephrine reuptake inhibitor. *Half-life after oral administration. *Italicized* represents $t_{1/2}$ of active metabolite. ^CYP: Cytochrome, UGT-G: UDP-glucuronosyltransferase-Glucuronidation.

Table 9 describes various pharmacokinetic profiles of monoamine oxidase inhibitors (MAOIs) and other miscellaneous drugs including mechanism of action (MOA), half-life (T$_{1/2}$) and metabolizing/inhibited enzymes:

Drug	MOA[#]	T$_{1/2}$ (Hours)*	Metabolism^	Enzyme Inhibited
Isocarboxazid[R,H]	MAOI	2.5	Not well understood	N/A
Phenelzine[R,H]	MAOI	11.6	Not well understood	N/A
Selegiline	MAOI	18-25	2B6, 2C9 and 3A4/5	Inhibitory action clinically not significant
Tranylcypromine [R,H]	MAOI	1.5-3.5	Not well understood	N/A
Bupropion[R,H]	DNRI	IR: 14 (8-24) SR/ER: 21; *20-37*	2D6, 2B6	Moderate 2D6
Nefazodone[H]	5HT2 Antag	2-4; *4-8*	3A4	Potent 3A4
Trazodone[H]	5HT2 Antag	IR: 7 ER: 10	2D6, 3A4	N/A
Vilazodone	Misc	25	3A4, 2C19, 2D6	Mod 2C19
Vortioxetine[R,H]	Misc	66	2D6, 3A4/5, 2C19, 2A6, 2C8, 2B6	N/A

[H] Caution advised/adjust in hepatic impairment
[R] Caution advised/adjust in renal impairment
[#]5HT2 Antag: serotonin receptor 2 antagonist, DNRI: dopamine norepinephrine reuptake inhibitor, MAOI: monoamine oxidase inhibitor, Misc: miscellaneous, SSRI: selective serotonin reuptake inhibitor. SNRI-serotonin norepinephrine reuptake inhibitor, TCA: tricyclic antidepressant. *Half-life after oral administration. *Italicized* represents t$_{1/2}$ of active metabolite. ^CYP: Cytochrome, UGT-G: UDP-glucuronosyltransferase-Glucuronidation.

Table 10 describes FDA approved indications for various drugs:

Drugs	FDA Approved Indications							
	GAD	MDD	OCD	PD	PMDD	PTSD	Social Phobia	Misc.
TCAs (SEE PEARLS)		X						
MAOIs		X						
Citalopram		X						
Escitalopram	X	X						
Fluoxetine		X	X	X	X			Bulimia Nervosa
Fluvoxamine			X					
Paroxetine	X	X	X	X	X	X	X	Hot Flashes; Menopause
Sertraline		X	X	X	X	X	X	
Desvenlafaxine		X						
Duloxetine	X	X						Diabetic Neuropathy FM; OA; MP
Levomilnacipran		X						
Milnacipran								FM
Venlafaxine	X	X		X			X	
Bupropion		X						Nicotine w/d; SAD
Nefazodone		X						
Trazodone		X						
Mirtazapine		X						
Vilazodone		X						
Vortioxetine		X						

DN: Diabetic Neuropathy, FM: Fibromyalgia, GAD: Generalized Anxiety Disorder, MDD: Major Depressive Disorder, MP: Musculoskeletal Pain, OA: Osteoarthritis, OCD: Obsessive Compulsive Disorder, PD: Panic Disorder, PMDD: Premenstrual Dysphoric Disorder, PTSD: Post Traumatic Stress Disorder, SAD: Seasonal affective disorder

Clinical Pearls

FDA March 2004--ALL antidepressants carry Black Box Warning (BBW) regarding suicidal thoughts and behaviors in children, adolescents and young adults (up to age 24.)[18,71]

FDA July 2014--ALL antidepressants carry warning regarding angle closure glaucoma.[19]

Cautious use of Tamoxifen with ADs with CYP2D6 inhibition (Paroxetine, Fluoxetine, Fluvoxamine, Duloxetine, Sertraline)[73-75]

Tricyclic Antidepressants (TCAs) [20-31]

<u>Mechanism of Action</u>: Inhibit reuptake of presynaptic 5HT and NE in addition to antagonism of histamine, alpha and muscarinic receptors (varying affinities per individual TCA). *Also known as "dirty SNRI".*

- Tertiary amines (amitriptyline, clomipramine, doxepin, imipramine, trimipramine) are more selective for serotonin than norepinephrine.
- Secondary amines (amoxapine, desipramine, maprotiline, nortriptyline, protriptyline) are more selective for norepinephrine than serotonin and are typically better tolerated.

<u>Adverse Effects</u>: Anticholinergic effects (blurred vision, cognitive impairment, constipation, urinary retention, xerostomia, etc.) cardiac effects (arrhythmias, hypotension/orthostasis, QT prolongation, tachycardia, etc.) dizziness, drowsiness, seizures, sexual dysfunction, toxicity, weight gain.

<u>Contraindications</u>: Acute myocardial infarction, carbamazepine hypersensitivity (similar tricyclic ring) or TCA hypersensitivity, MAOI within 14 days.

<u>FDA approved indications</u>:
- Depression (**EXCEPT** Clomipramine)
- OCD (Clomipramine)
- Anxiety/Insomnia/Pruritus (Doxepin)
- Enuresis (Imipramine)

<u>Other Clinical Pearls</u>:
- **TCAs CAN BE TOXIC IN OVERDOSE—CAUTION IN SUICIDAL PATIENTS**
- **Caution in hepatic impairment—lower initial dose & titration**
- CYP2D6 Inhibitors can alter hepatic metabolism of TCAs increasing adverse events: *Cimetidine may increase TCAs by 50%--hepatic metabolism inhibition*
- Barbiturates, alcohol and other CNS depressants can increase CNS depression and drowsiness
- TCAs are often taken at bedtime due to sedation
- Multiple off label uses: enuresis, fibromyalgia, insomnia, migraine prophylaxis, neuropathic pain, overactive bladder, panic disorder, etc.
- Amoxapine- metabolite of Loxapine (D2 antagonist-watch for extrapyramidal symptoms)
- Amitriptyline- Similar chemical structure to Cyclobenzaprine
- Amitriptyline metabolizes to Nortriptyline
- Imipramine-metabolizes to Desipramine
- Doxepin's antihistaminic potency ~ 800 times greater than that of diphenhydramine (hence it's use in pruritus, chronic urticaria and cream)[79,80]

<u>Monitoring serum concentrations</u>:
Levels are drawn as trough values just before next dose and should include both tertiary and secondary metabolites[14]

Drug	Serum Therapeutic Concentration
Amitriptyline	100-250 ng/mL or mcg/L
Clomipramine	50-250 ng/mL or mcg/L
Desclomipramine	150-350 ng/mL or mcg/L
Clomipramine + Desmethyl Total	200-600 ng/mL or mcg/L
Desipramine	50-300 ng/mL or mcg/L
Doxepin	30-150 ng/mL or mcg/L
Imipramine	150-250 ng/mL or mcg/L
Nortriptyline	50–150 ng/ml or mcg/L
Amitriptyline + Nortriptyline Total	100-200 ng/mL or mcg/L

- Labs levels may vary slightly depending upon lab device used
- Toxicity of TCAs is primarily anticholinergic and cardiovascular
- Increased incidence of anticholinergic adverse events is associated with plasma TCA concentrations >500 mg/L though may be experienced at lower plasma TCA concentrations [11]
- Lethal cardiotoxicity has been associated with plasma TCA concentrations >1000 mg/L and a QRS duration of >100 ms [12,13]

Monoamine Oxidase Inhibitors (MAOIs)

Mechanism of Action: Inhibit monoamine oxidase (MAO) irreversibly. MAO-A metabolizes 5HT and NE (responsible for antidepressant effects). MAO-B metabolizes trace amines. MAO-A & MAO-B both metabolize dopamine and tyramine. Takes up to 2 weeks to replenish MAO enzyme after medication discontinuation (hence medication washout recommendations).

Adverse Effects: Anticholinergic effects, hypotension, hypertensive crisis (tyramine containing foods/drinks and sympathomimetic medications), sedation (phenelzine), insomnia/stimulation (selegiline-amphetamine metabolite & tranylcypromine-structurally similar to amphetamine), sexual dysfunction.

Contraindications: Children, pheochromocytoma, surgery (should discontinue 10 days prior to elective surgery). Concurrent use of sympathomimetics, serotonergic agents, or tyramine containing foods. Tyramine is an amino acid that helps regulate blood pressure. It's naturally occurring in the body and also in certain foods. MAOIs block an enzyme that breaks down excess tyramine. Excessive tyramine can cause serious spikes in blood pressure, also known as hypertensive crisis.

Foods that Contain Tyramine:
- All tap beers (including homemade bottled/canned beers)
- Strong or Aged cheeses (aged cheddar, blue cheeses, brie, camembert, parmesan and swiss)
- Aged, smoked and processed meats (bacon, bologna, corned beef, hot dogs, jerky, pepperoni, salami, sausages, smoked fish)
- Fermented and pickled foods (sauerkraut, caviar, tofu, pickles)
- Dried/overripe fruits (avocados, overripe bananas, raisins and prunes)
- Soybeans/soybean products, fava beans and other broad bean pods

- Red and white wine (chianti, vermouth, etc)
- Yeast extracts (brewer's yeast, marmite and sour dough bread)
- Spoiled or improperly stored food of any kind

> **SERIOUS INTERACTIONS (DRUG-DRUG & DRUG-FOOD):**
> **AVOID TYRAMINE-CONTAINING FOODS**[16]

Approximate MAOI Dose Equivalency:
40 mg isocarboxazid = 20 mg tranylcypromine = 45 mg phenelzine [15]

Isocarboxazid (Marplan®)[62]
Available: 10 mg tablets
Dose: 20-60 mg/day (BID-QID)
Renal: *Caution in mild-mod renal impairment; contraindicated in severe renal impairment*
Hepatic: *Contraindicated* in patients with abnormal liver function tests, hepatic impairment or history of liver disease

Phenelzine (Nardil®)[63]
Available: 15 mg tablets
Dose: Typically initiated at 15 mg once daily and further titrated up to 45-90 mg/day divided three to four times a day
Renal: *Caution in mild-mod renal impairment; contraindicated in severe renal impairment*
Hepatic: *Contraindicated* in patients with abnormal liver function tests, hepatic impairment or history of liver disease
- More weight gain, sedation and sexual dysfunction when compared to Tranylcypromine.

Selegiline (EMSAM®)[64,76]
Available: 6, 9, 12 mg patches; dose 6-12 mg/24 hr
Alternative forms/dosing not discussed as not indicated for AD treatment
Dose: Initiate at 6 mg/24 hr may titrate by 3 mg/24hr up to 12 mg/24 hr
Renal: No adjustment
Hepatic: No adjustment
- No dietary restriction with 6mg/24 hr dose; unrestricted dietary tyramine data in clinical trials limited at 9 or 12mg/24 hr so dietary restrictions should be followed at these doses.
- Tends to be stimulating; metabolizes to amphetamine.
- Direct inhibition of MAO-A in GI tract is avoided with transdermal use.
- Selegiline is selective MAO-B inhibitor at low doses though lacks AD properties at low doses and primarily used in treatment of Parkinson disease.

Tranylcypromine (Parnate®)[65]

Dose: typically initiated at 10 mg once daily and further titrated up to 30-60 mg/day.

Renal: *Caution in mild-mod renal impairment; contraindicated in severe renal impairment.*

Hepatic: *Contraindicated* in patients with abnormal LFTs, hepatic impairment or history of liver disease.

- Similar chemical structure to amphetamines; some stimulant properties.
- Tends to be activating; last dose should be given in early afternoon.
- Less likely than Phenelzine to cause weight gain.

Selective Serotonin Reuptake Inhibitors (SSRIs)

MOA: Selective serotonin reuptake inhibition. Increase neural concentrations of serotonin by blocking reuptake of serotonin into the presynaptic cell. This results in increased serotonin in the synapse available for binding to postsynaptic receptors.

Adverse Effects: anxiety, diarrhea, headache, insomnia, nausea, QT prolongation (see below), sexual dysfunction, sweating, weight loss.

Contraindications: MAOIs within 14 days.

Approximate SSRI Dose Equivalency:
Escitalopram 10 mg = Citalopram 20 mg = Fluoxetine 20 mg = Paroxetine 20 mg (CR 25 mg) = Sertraline 50 mg = Fluvoxamine 100 mg.

Citalopram (Celexa®)[32]

Dose: 10-40 mg; Max 20 mg/day in elderly (greater than 60 years of age) or if receiving potent CYP2C19 inhibitors (Cimetidine, Omeprazole, etc).

Renal: No adjustment mild-mod impairment; *caution* advised in severe impairment.

Hepatic: Max: 20 mg/day

- Dose-related QT prolongation: 8.5 msec/20 mg; 12.6 msec/40 mg; 18.5 msec/60 mg. Discontinue if QTc >500 msec.
- Monitor EKG in patients with heart failure or other known medications known to prolong QT interval.
- Relatively low drug-drug interaction potential.

Escitalopram (Lexapro®)[33]

Dose: 5-20mg/day; Max of 10mg/day in elderly.

Renal: No adjustment mild-mod impairment; *caution* advised in severe impairment.

Hepatic: Max: 10 mg/day.

- Enantiomer (S isomer) of Citalopram (~2 times as potent).
- Tends to be better tolerated/less AE/less DI than Citalopram.
- Relatively low drug-drug interaction potential.

Fluoxetine (Prozac®/Weekly™; Sarafem®; Selfemra®)[40-42]

Available: 10, 20, 40 mg capsules; 90 mg DR capsule; 20 mg/5mL oral solution; 10, 15, 20, 40, 60 mg tablets

Dose: 10-80 mg/day.

Renal: No adjustment.

Hepatic: *Adjust*/decrease dose or frequency.

- **POTENT CYP 2D6 INHIBITOR.**
- LONG half-life of 4-6 days; Active Metabolite of 7-9.3 days.
- Usually AM dosing as tends to be activating; may cause insomnia.
- Less likely to cause antidepressant discontinuation syndrome.
- Highly protein bound (95%).

Fluvoxamine (Luvox®/CR®)[34]

Available: 25, 50, 100 mg tablets; 100, 150 mg ER capsules

Dose: 25-300 mg/day (usually HS). (HS due to sedation)

Renal: No adjustment.

Hepatic: Titrate slowly.

- FDA approved for OCD not MDD.
- **POTENT CYP 1A2, 2C19 & MODERATE 3A4 INHIBITOR.**

Paroxetine (Brisdelle®; Paxil®/CR®; Pexeva®)[35-39]

Available: 10, 20, 30, 40 mg tablets; 10 mg/5mL oral suspension; 12.5, 25, 37.5 mg CR tablets; 7.5 mg capsule

Dose: 10-60 mg/day (usually PM or HS due to sedation)

Renal: *CrCl < 30 mL/min:* start with 10 mg/day; Max 40 mg/day

Hepatic: *Severe impairment:* start with 10 mg/day; Max 40 mg/day

- **POTENT CYP 2D6 INHIBITOR**
- Of SSRIs: strong anticholinergic, most sedating, sexual dysfunction and discontinuation syndrome more common, most likely to cause weight gain (~25% gain >7% of their body weight)
- Only SSRI without warning of QT prolongation per PI and article[72]
- Highest rate of sexual dysfunction [81,82]
- Highly protein bound (93-95%)

Sertraline (Zoloft®)[43]

Available: 25, 50, 100 mg tablets; 20 mg/mL oral solution

Dose: 25-200 mg/day.

Renal: No adjustment.

Hepatic: Suggested to decrease dose or frequency.

- Diarrhea more common (~8%) adverse reaction compared to other SSRIs.
- Usually AM dosing to minimize insomnia.
- Highly protein bound (98%).
- Relatively low drug-drug interaction potential.

Serotonin Norepinephrine Reuptake Inhibitors (SNRIs)

<u>MOA:</u> Serotonin and Norepinephrine Reuptake Inhibition. Increase neural concentrations of serotonin and norepinephrine by blocking reuptake into the presynaptic neuron. This results in increased serotonin and norepinephrine in the synapse available for binding to postsynaptic receptors.

<u>Adverse Effects:</u> Constipation, diaphoresis, dizziness, headache, hypertension, insomnia, nausea, sexual dysfunction

<u>Contraindications:</u> MAOIs within 14 days, monitor in hepatic and renal impairment, caution in uncontrolled narrow angle glaucoma

<u>Approximate dose equivalency:</u>[77,78]

Duloxetine 30 mg = Venlafaxine 75 mg = Desvenlafaxine 50 mg

Desvenlafaxine (Khedezla®; Pristiq®)[48,49]

Available: 25, 50, 100 mg ER tablets

<u>Dose:</u> 50-100 mg/day; studied up to 400 mg/day; manufacturer claims no additional benefit >50 mg/day.

<u>Renal:</u> *CrCl 30-50 mL/min:* maximum of 50 mg/day. *CrCl < 30 mL/min:* maximum of 50 mg every other day.

<u>Hepatic:</u> *Moderate to severe impairment* 50 mg daily with max of 100 mg/day.

- **Do not crush/cut/chew tablet. Potential for ghost tablet.**
- Monitor for increase in blood pressure

Duloxetine (Cymbalta®; Irenka®)[46,47]

Available: 20, 30, 40, 60 mg DR capsules

<u>Dose:</u> 30-120 mg/day.

<u>Renal:</u> Avoid if *CrCl < 30 mL/min.*

<u>Hepatic:</u> *Avoid* in patients with hepatic impairment or heavy alcohol use.

- Similarly balanced ("du" *dual*) affinity for 5HT and NE transporters
- Higher incidence of dose related constipation and dry mouth; antagonizes M1 muscarinic receptors to greater degree than Venlafaxine
- Contraindicated with uncontrolled narrow angle glaucoma
- Highly protein bound (>90%)

Levomilnacipran (Fetzima®)[50]

Available: 20, 40, 80, 120 mg ER capsules

<u>Dose:</u> 40-120 mg/day.

<u>Renal:</u> *CrCl 30-59 mL/min:* maximum of 80 mg/day. *CrCl 15-29 mL/min:* maximum of 40 mg/day. *CrCl <15 mL/mi:* -DO NOT USE.

<u>Hepatic:</u> No adjustment.

- **NE > 5HT**; Greater affinity for NE compared to 5HT transporters.
- Monitor for increases in blood pressure.
- Contraindicated with uncontrolled narrow angle glaucoma.

Milnacipran (Savella®)[51]

Available: 12.5, 25, 50, 100 mg tablets

Dose: 50 mg BID; maximum 200 mg/day

Renal: *CrCl 30-49 mL/min*: caution advised. *CrCl 5-29mL/min*: decrease dose by 50%. Max: 100 mg/day

Hepatic: *Severe impairment caution* advised; chronic hepatic disease-avoid

- Not FDA indicated for MDD ONLY Fibromyalgia
- NE > 5HT; affinity for NE over 5HT inhibition by ~3-fold

Venlafaxine (Effexor®/XR®)[44,45]

Available: 25, 37.5, 50, 75, 100 mg IR tablets; 37.5, 75, 150 mg ER capsules; 37.5, 75, 150, 225 mg ER tablets

Dose: **IR:** 75-375 mg/day in divided dose. **ER/XR:** 75-225 mg/day.

Renal: *CrCl 10-70 mL/min:* decrease dose 25-50%. *CrCl <10 mL/min*: decrease dose 50%.

Hepatic: *Mild-mod impairment*: decrease 50%.

- 5HT > NE at lower doses (<150 mg/day)
- Inhibits DA transporters at dose > 450 mg/day
- Monitor for increase in blood pressure; dose related hypertension
- Greater NE affinity at doses > 150 mg/day
- Higher rates nausea, sexual dysfunction and antidepressant discontinuation syndrome
- Taper dose no more than 75 mg/week to discontinue.
- **May open ER capsule BUT Do Not Cut/Crush/Chew/Dissolve Contents**
- **Do not crush/cut/chew tablet. Potential for ghost tablet.**

Alpha 2 Antagonist + 5HT2 & 5HT3 Antagonist

MOA: Enhance central noradrenergic and serotonergic activity via indirect alpha 2 antagonism. Additionally, blocks 5HT2 & 5HT3 post-synaptic receptors, strong H1 antagonist and weak M1 & alpha 1 antagonist.

Adverse Effects: dizziness, drowsiness, increased appetite, increased cholesterol, weight gain

Contraindications: History of hypersensitivity, MAOIs within 14 days

Mirtazapine (Remeron®/SolTab®)[66,67]

Available: 7.5, 15, 30, 45mg tablets; 15, 30, 45 mg ODT

Dose: 15-45 mg at bedtime.

Renal: *CrCl 11-39 mL/min:* ~30% reduction in clearance. *CrCl <10 mL/min:* ~50% reduction in clearance.

Hepatic: *Caution* advised; clearance decreased by 30%.

- Not associated with sexual dysfunction compared to other antidepressants.
- Helpful for those with poor appetite; associated with weight gain.
- Monitor cholesterol/triglycerides (potential to increase).

- Dosed at HS due to sedation.
- Anxiolytic & antiemetic properties d/t respective 5HT2 & 5HT3 blockade.
- Faster antidepressant onset of action compared to other antidepressants.[2]
- Rare neutropenia & leukopenia (~0.1%).

Serotonin 2 Antagonists

MOA: Blockade of postsynaptic (5HT2) receptors with additional inhibition of pre-synaptic 5HT receptors.
Adverse Effects: Constipation, dizziness, drowsiness, dry mouth, headache, orthostatic hypotension.
Contraindications: MAOIs within 14 days (see hepatic info for Nefazodone).

Nefazodone (Serzone®)[61]
Available: 50, 100, 150, 200, 250 mg tablets
Dose: 150-300 mg BID; start 100 mg BID.
Renal: No adjustment.
Hepatic: *Contraindicated* in acute hepatic disease or elevated LFTs.
- **STRONG CYP 3A4 INHIBITOR.**
- Increase various (3A4) statin levels/increase risk of rhabdomyolysis.
- May increase central nervous system depressant effects of various (3A4) benzodiazepines.
- Associated with liver failure in some patients; monitor liver function tests.
  - 1 per 250,000-300,000 patient years.
- Not associated with sexual dysfunction compared to other antidepressants.
- Highly protein bound (99%).
- Possess m-chlorophenylpiperazine (mCPP) metabolite like Trazodone.

Trazodone (Desyrel®; Oleptro®)[59,60]
Available: 50, 100, 150, 300 mg tablets; 150, 300 mg ER capsules
Dose: 50-100 mg BID-TID; Max 400 mg/day outpatient; Max 600 mg/day inpatient;
Insomnia: 25-200 mg HS.
Renal: No adjustment
Hepatic: Caution advised
- Linked to rare condition called priapism
- Seek emergency treatment if erection last more than 4 hours
- Weak antidepressant at low doses; used for insomnia at low doses
- Antidepressant activity typically not seen until >150 mg
- Not associated with sexual dysfunction compared to other antidepressants.
- Active metabolite mCPP (m-chlorophenylpiperazine) may trigger a migraine headache

Dopamine + Norepinephrine Reuptake Inhibitor (DNRI)

<u>MOA:</u> Weak inhibition of norepinephrine along with dopamine reuptake into the presynaptic neuron resulting in increases of neuronal concentrations in the synapse. This results in increased dopamine and norepinephrine in the synapse available for binding to postsynaptic receptors.

<u>Adverse Effects:</u> abnormal dreams, agitation, anxiety, headache, insomnia, nausea, seizures, tachycardia, weight loss

<u>Contraindications:</u> History of hypersensitivity, MAOIs, alcohol withdrawal, eating disorders, seizure disorder

Bupropion (Aplenzin®; Buproban®; Forfivo XL®;Wellbutrin®/SR®/XL®; Zyban®)[52-58]

Available: HCl (hydrochloride salt) 75, 100 mg IR tablets; 100, 150, 200 mg SR tablets; 150, 300, 450 mg ER/XL tablets; HBr (hydrobromide salt) 174, 348, 522 mg ER tablets (equate to HCl 150, 300, 450 mg dose respectively)

<u>Dose:</u> **IR:** 100 mg BID-TID; Max single dose 150 mg; Max daily dose: 450 mg.
SR: 150 mg QAM-BID; Max single dose 200 mg; Max daily dose: 400 mg.
ER/XL: 150-450 mg once daily; Max single & daily dose: 450 mg.
<u>Renal Dose:</u> Consider dose/frequency reduction.
<u>Hepatic Dose:</u> Consider dose/frequency reduction (Child-Pugh Class A) 100 mg/day or 150 mg Q48H (Child-Pugh Class B or C).

- Good choice for patients with low energy caused by depression
- May titrate up after 3-4 days
- Useful for smoking cessation
- Common augmenting agent
- Should not be taken too late in the day due to insomnia
- Not associated with sexual side effects & weight gain (compared to other antidepressants)

Miscellaneous Antidepressants- SSRI + 5HT1A Partial Agonist

<u>MOA:</u> SSRI + 5HT1A partial agonism
<u>Adverse Effects:</u> abnormal dreams, diarrhea, dizziness, insomnia, nausea, restlessness, vomiting, xerostomia
<u>Contraindications:</u> History of hypersensitivity, MAOIs within 14 days

Vilazodone (Viibryd®)[68]

Available: 10, 20, 40 mg tablets
<u>Dose:</u> 20-40 mg daily; initiate 10 mg daily for 7days.
<u>Renal:</u> No adjustment
<u>Hepatic:</u> No adjustment

- Do not adjust dose more frequently than every 7 days
- Highly protein bound (96-99%).
- Take with food to enhance bioavailability + minimize GI distress
  Plasma concentrations decreased by 50% in fasting state.

Serotonin Modulators

<u>MOA:</u> SSRI + 5HT1A Agonist + 5HT3 Antagonist (Additional 5HT1B Partial Agonist + 5HT1D & 5HT7 Antagonist)

<u>Adverse Effects:</u> constipation, nausea, vomiting, sexual dysfunction

<u>Contraindications:</u> History of hypersensitivity, MAOIs within 14 days

Vortioxetine (Trintellix®)[69]

Available: 5, 10, 20 mg tablets

<u>Dose:</u> 10-20 mg daily; Max of 10 mg/day in CYP2D6 poor metabolizers

<u>Renal:</u> No adjustment

<u>Hepatic:</u> Mild-mod impairment-no adjustment; Severe impairment-*caution*

- Sexual dysfunction may be less than SSRIs
- May aid in cognitive complaints (reduced concentration, forgetfulness, etc)
- FDA issued brand name change--confusion between the antidepressant *Brintellix* (vortioxetine) and the antiplatelet medication *Brilinta®* (ticagrelor)[70]
- Highly protein bound (98%)

Atypical Antipsychotics for MDD Adjunctive Treatment
Dosing below is specific to antidepressant treatment

Aripiprazole (Abilify/Discmelt®; Abilify Maintena®)[84-87]

Available: 2, 5, 10, 15, 20, 30 mg tablets; 10, 15 mg ODT; 1 mg/mL Oral Solution; 9.75 mg/1.3 mL short acting IM injection; 300, 400 mg suspension for long-acting injectable

<u>Dose:</u> 2-5 mg DAILY (PO adjunctive therapy). Adjust dose at 5 mg intervals of no less than 1 week each. Dose range 2-15 mg/day. Max 15 mg/day (MDD adjunct) or 30 mg/day for other conditions.

<u>Renal:</u> No adjustment necessary

<u>Hepatic:</u> No adjustment necessary

- Long half-life--no need to dose more than QDAILY; Steady state reached in ~ 2 weeks
- Warnings of new onset impulse-control issues
- Dosage adjustment with concurrent CYP450 inducer/inhibitor: does not apply when used for adjunctive therapy for major depressive disorder.

Olanzapine + Fluoxetine (Symbyax®)[90]

Available: 3/25, 6/25, 6/50, 12/25, 12/50 mg capsules
Dose: 6/25 mg/day and adjust dose if indicated/tolerated. Max Dose: 18/75 mg
Renal: No dose adjustment
Hepatic: Initially 3/25 mg increased as tolerated
- For acute and maintenance of treatment-resistant depression

Approximate Dose Equivalency:

Symbyax® 3/25 mg	Symbyax® 6/25 mg	Symbyax® 12/25 mg	Symbyax® 6/50 mg	Symbyax® 12/50 mg
Olanzapine 2.5mg + Fluoxetine 20mg	Olanzapine 5mg + Fluoxetine 20mg	Olanzapine 12.5mg + Fluoxetine 20mg	Olanzapine 5mg + Fluoxetine 50mg	Olanzapine 12.5mg + Fluoxetine 50mg

Quetiapine (Seroquel®; Seroquel XR®)[89-89]

Available: 25, 50, 100, 200, 300, 400 mg tablets; 50, 150, 200, 300, 400 mg Extended Release Tablets
Dose: **XR tablets:** 50 mg in the evening on day 1 and day 2 then increase to 150 mg in the evening. Dose range for 150-300 mg/day for MDD. Up to 800 mg/day other conditions.
Renal: No dose adjustment needed with CrCl > 10 mL/min
Hepatic: Hepatic impairment results in 30% reduced clearance
- Usually dose at bedtime due to sedation
- Slow titration in patients with risk of hypotension
- If off for > 1 week follow initial titration
- REDUCE DOSE 1/6th OF ORIGINAL DOSE WITH POTENT 3A4 INHBITORS
- MAY NEED TO INCREASE DOSE 5-FOLD WITH POTENT 3A4 INDUCERS
- XR version had statistically significant increases in Cmax & AUC with high-fat meal (800-1000 calories) but no significant effect with light meal of 300 calories. XR should be given WITHOUT FOOD or LIGHT MEAL ONLY.

Antipsychotics

Antipsychotics are used for various psychiatric conditions, including schizophrenia, psychosis, bipolar disorder, and agitation. The older antipsychotics are also known as first generation antipsychotics (FGA), or typical antipsychotics. These agents have high affinity for dopamine D_2 receptors. The newer antipsychotics are also known as second generation antipsychotics (SGA), or atypical antipsychotics. These agents have lower affinity for D_2 receptors, but have greater affinity for serotonin $5\text{-}HT_2$ receptors.[1]

All antipsychotics have a black box warning regarding increased risk of death in elderly patients with dementia related psychosis
In February 2017, FDA approved updates to all antipsychotic medication labels to warn of somnolence, postural hypotension, and motor and sensory instability risks, which could lead to falls and subsequent fractures or other injuries.

This section includes:
- Hypothesis for use of antipsychotics
- Various adverse reactions associated with antipsychotics
- Diagnostic criteria of schizophrenia, schizoaffective disorder, schizophreniform disorder, and bipolar disorder
- Overview of first and second generation antipsychotics
- Details of first and second generation antipsychotics

Dopamine Hypothesis[1]

The therapeutic effects of antipsychotics in patients with schizophrenia supports the dopamine hypothesis. This hypothesis suggests that the disorder is due to excess dopamine activity in the brain. However, this hypothesis does not fully explain the pathogenesis of schizophrenia, as antipsychotics only partially treats symptoms. Moreover, drugs with higher affinity for other receptors than dopamine receptors are effective in patients with schizophrenia. Other receptors that are thought to have antipsychotic effects include various serotonin receptors ($5\text{-}HT_{1, 2, 2A, 1D}$), and α_1 adrenergic receptor. Many of these receptors are mainly targeted by second generation antipsychotics.

Adverse Reactions

Extrapyramidal side effects (EPS)[1]

Antipsychotics, especially drugs that have high affinity for dopamine receptors, have extrapyramidal side effects (EPS). Drugs with low-potency for dopamine receptors have lower risk for EPS. Extrapyramidal side effects include Parkinson-like syndrome with bradykinesia, rigidity, tremor, and acute dystonic reaction are thought to be dose-dependent.

Tardive Dyskinesias (TD)[1]
Tardive Dyskinesia usually develop after several years of antipsychotic drug therapy. It is thought to be caused by dopamine receptor sensitization.

Endocrine and Metabolic Effects[1]
Hyperprolactinemia, gynecomastia, and amenorrhea-galactorrhea syndrome are seen with antipsychotics. These side effects are more pronounced with first generation antipsychotics, as these are more selective for dopamine receptors. Of the atypical antipsychotics, elevated prolactin is most common with risperidone. As these agents block dopamine D_2 receptors in the pituitary, the inhibitory regulator of prolactin secretion becomes absent. This results in elevated prolactin levels. Increase in weight and hyperglycemia are common with atypicals, especially with clozapine, olanzapine, and quetiapine.

Neuroleptic Malignant Syndrome[1]
Neuroleptic malignant syndrome may be a life-threatening condition. It is more prevalent in patients who are sensitive to the extrapyramidal effects of antipsychotics. Symptoms include muscle rigidity, impairment of sweating, hyperpyrexia, and autonomic instability. Diazepam, dantrolene, and dopamine agonists are often used to treat neuroleptic malignant syndrome.

DIAGNOSTIC CRITERIA (DSM-5)[2]

Schizophrenia
A. Two or more of the characteristic symptoms below are present for a significant portion of time during one-month period. At least one must be (1), (2), or (3):
1. Delusions
2. Hallucinations
3. Disorganized speech (e.g., frequent derailment or incoherence)
4. Grossly disorganized or catatonic behavior
5. Negative symptoms

B. For a significant portion of the time since the onset of the disturbance, level of functioning in one or more major areas, such as work, interpersonal relations, or self-care, is markedly below the level achieved prior to onset.

C. Continuous signs of the disturbance persist for at least 6 months. This 6-month period must include at least one month of symptoms (or less if successfully treated) that meets criterion A and may include periods of prodromal or residual symptoms. During these prodromal or residual periods, the signs of the disturbance may be manifested by only negative symptoms or by two or more symptoms listed in Criterion A present in an attenuated form (e.g., odd beliefs, unusual perceptual experiences).

D. Schizoaffective disorder and depressive or bipolar disorder with psychotic features have been ruled out because either 1) no major depressive or manic episodes have occurred concurrently with the active-phase symptoms, or 2) if mood episodes have occurred during active-phase symptoms, they have been present for a minority of the total duration of the active and residual periods of the illness.

E. The disturbance is not attributable to the physiological effects of a substance (e.g., a drug of abuse, a medication) or another medical condition

F. If there is a history of autism spectrum disorder or a communication disorder of childhood onset, the additional diagnosis of schizophrenia is made only if prominent delusions or hallucinations, in addition to the other required symptoms of schizophrenia, are also present for at least 1 month (or less if successfully treated).

> Diagnostic features of schizophrenia include:
> - Positive symptoms (features patient have that are normally not present): delusions, hallucinations, disorganized speech, grossly abnormal psychomotor behavior, including catatonia.
> - Negative symptoms (features patient does not have that are normally present): diminished emotional expression, avolition, alogia, anhedonia, asociality.

Schizoaffective Disorder

A. An uninterrupted period of illness during which there is a major mood episode (major depressive or manic) concurrent with Criterion A of schizophrenia.

B. Delusions or hallucinations for 2 or more weeks in the absence of a major mood episode (depressive or manic) during the lifetime duration of the illness.

C. Symptoms that meet criteria for a major mood episode are present for the majority of the total duration of the active and residual potions of the illness.

D. The disturbance is not attributable to the effects of a substance (e.g., a drug of abuse, a medication) or another medical condition.

Schizophreniform Disorder

A. Two or more of the following, each present for a significant portion of time during a 1-month period (or less if successfully treated). At least one of these must be (1), (2), or (3):
    1. Delusions
    2. Hallucinations
    3. Disorganized speech (e.g., frequent derailment or incoherence)
    4. Grossly disorganized or catatonic behavior
    5. Negative symptoms (i.e. diminished emotional expression or avolition)

B. An episode of the disorder lasts at least one month but less than 6 months. When the diagnosis must be made without waiting for recovery, it should be qualified as "provisional."

C. Schizoaffective disorder and depressive or bipolar disorder with psychotic features have been ruled out because either 1) no major depressive or manic

episodes have occurred concurrently with the active-phase symptoms, or 2) if mood episodes have occurred during active-phase symptoms, they have been present for a minority of the total duration of the active and residual periods of the illness.
D. The disturbance is not attributable to the physiological effects of a substance (e.g., a drug of abuse, a medication) or another medical condition.

Brief Psychotic Disorder
A. Presence of one (or more) of the following symptoms. At least one of these must be (1), (2), or (3):
    1. Delusions
    2. Hallucinations
    3. Disorganized speech
    4. Grossly disorganized or catatonic behavior
B. Duration of an episode of the disturbance is at least 1 day but less than 1 month, with eventual full return to premorbid level of functioning
C. The disturbance is not better explained by major depressive or bipolar disorder with psychotic features or another psychotic disorder such as schizophrenia or catatonia, and is not attributable to the physiological effects of a substance (e.g., a drug of abuse, a medication) or another medical condition.

Diagnostic criteria for bipolar disorder is discussed in the "Bipolar Disorder, Antiepileptic Drugs & Mood Stabilizers" section.

Table 1 describes classification of typical antipsychotic drugs, also known as first generation antipsychotics (FGA).[1,3]

Classification	Drug
Phenothiazines	Chlorpromazine, Thioridazine, Fluphenazine, Perphenazine, Prochlorperazine, Trifluoperazine
Thioxanthenes	Thiothixene
Butyrophenones	Haloperidol, Droperidol

Table 2 describes dosage form, route of administration, and usual daily dose of typical antipsychotics (first generation antipsychotics): [3-18, 43-45]

Generic Name	Brand Name	Dosage Form*	Route#	Dose Range
Chlorprom-azine	Thorazine®	SI, T	PO, IV, IM	PO: 30 – 800 mg divided 2-4x/day IV/IM: 25-50 mg
Droperidol	Inapsine®	SI	IV, IM	IM/IV: 2.5-5 mg
Fluphenazine	Prolixin®	OC, SI (HCl), T, OE, LAI (deca-noate)	IM, PO, SubQ	PO: 2.5-20mg/day in 3-4 divided doses IM (HCl): 1.25-10 mg/day divided q6-8 hour interval IM/SubQ: 12.5-25 mg q3-4 weeks
Haloperidol	Haldol®	OC, SI (lactate) PO, LAI (deca-noate)	IM, PO	PO: 0.5 – 5 mg BID-TID IM (lactate): 5 – 10 mg q4-6 hours IM (decanoate): 50 – 200 mg every 4 weeks
Molindone	Moban®	T	PO	50-225mg/day in 3-4 divided doses
Perphenazine	Trilafon®	T	PO	4-16 mg 2-4x/day
Pimozide	Orap®	T	PO	0.5-2 mg/day divided
Prochlor-perazine	Compazine® Compro®	T, SI (edisy-late), RS	PO, IM, IV, PR	PO: 5-10 mg 3-4x/day IM (edisylate): 5-10 mg q3-4 hours IM/IV (edisylate): 5-10 mg IM q3-4 hours, 2.5-10 mg slow IV injection PR: 25 mg BID
Thioridazine	Mellaril®	T	PO	150-800 mg divided 2-4x/day
Thiothixene	Navane®	C	PO	6-30 mg/day in divided doses
Trifluo-perazine	Stelazine®	T	PO	2-20 mg/day divided

*SI: Solution for injection, T: tablet, OC : Concentrate solution for oral use, OE : Elixir for oral use, RS: Rectal Suppository, LAI: Long-acting injectable
#SubQ: Subcutaneously, PO: oral route, IM: intramuscularly, PR: per rectum

Table 3 describes various pharmacokinetic profiles of typical antipsychotics (first generation antipsychotics) including mechanism of action (MOA), half-life ($t_{1/2}$), and metabolizing/inhibited enzymes:[3-20, 63-73]

Drug	MOA[#]	$T_{1/2}$ (Hours)*	Metabolism^	Enzyme Inhibited^
Chlor-promazine[H, R]	Blocks dopamine and α-adrenergic receptors	~23-37	CYP 2D6	CYP2D6
Droperidol[H, R]	Blocks dopamine and α-adrenergic receptors	~2.3 hours	Hepatic	N/A
Fluphen-azine[H, R]	Blocks D_2 receptors	PO: 14.4 to 16.4 IM (decanoate): ~14 days	CYP2D6	CYPs 1A2, 2C9, 2E1, 2D6
Haloperidol	Blocks D_2 receptors	IM (decanoate): 21 days IM (Lactate): 20 hours PO: 14-37 hours	CYP3A4, 2D6, glucuro-nidation	CYP2D6
Molindone[H]	Blocks D_2 receptors	1.5	Hepatic	N/A
Perphen-azine[H, R]	Blocks D_2 receptors	9-12	CYPs 2D6, 3A4, 1A2, 2C9, 2C19	CYP1A2; CYP2D6
Pimozide[H, R]	Dopamine antagonist	55	3A4, 1A2, 2D6	CYP2E1, CYP2D6
Prochlor-perazine[H]	Blocks D_1, D_2, α-adrenergic, anti-cholinergic receptors	6.8-9	N/A	N/A
Thioridazine[H]	Blocks dopamine	21-24	CYPs 2C19, 2D6	CYPs 1A2, 2C9, 2D6, 2E1
Thiothixene[H]	Blocks dopamine	34	CYP1A2	N/A
Trifluo-perazine[H]	Blocks D_2 receptors	3-12	1A2	N/A

[H]Caution advised in hepatic impairment   [R]Caution advised in renal impairment
*After Oral Administration. ^CYP: Cytochrome

Table 4 describes FDA approved indications for typical antipsychotic drugs:[3-18]

Drugs	Bipolar Disorder	Psychosis	Schizo-phrenia	N/V[#]	Others*
Chlorpromazine	X	X	X	X	Intractable hiccups
Droperidol					PONV
Fluphenazine		X	X		
Haloperidol			X		Tourette's
Molindone			X		
Perphenazine			X	X	
Pimozide					Tourette's
Prochlorperazine			X	X	
Thioridazine			X		
Thiothixene			X		
Trifluoperazine			X		Non-psychotic anxiety
[#]N/V: Nausea/Vomiting; *PONV: Postoperative nausea/vomiting					

Clinical Pearls

First Generation Antipsychotics (FGAs)[3-18]

- First generation antipsychotics (typical antipsychotics) are thought to work by blocking the dopamine type 2 (D_2) receptors. It also targets alpha-adrenergic, serotonergic, histaminergic, and muscarinic receptors.
- FGAs may increase the risk of death in elderly patients with dementia-related psychosis, seizure disorder, neuroleptic malignant syndrome (NMS), and increased risk of tardive dyskinesia (TD) in the elderly, especially women.
- FGAs may increase risk of QT prolongation and torsades de pointes (TdP).
- Leukopenia/neutropenia and agranulocytosis have been reported temporally related to antipsychotic agents. Use with caution in patients with hematological disease.
- Prior to administration of long acting injectable, oral formulation must be given to establish tolerability.
- Caution in patients with seizure disorder, history of seizures, or with other conditions that may lower the seizure threshold.
- Antipsychotics can cause motor and sensory instability, which may lead to falls with potential for fractures and other injuries.
- FGAs may stimulate the release of prolactin and may induce infertility in either men or women, or may induce other endocrine abnormalities. Some breast cancers may be prolactin-dependent- FGAs should be used with extreme caution in patients with history of breast cancer.

Table 5 describes dosage form, route of administration, and usual daily dose of atypical antipsychotics (second generation antipsychotics): [23-39, 42, 52]

Generic Name	Brand Name	Dosage Form*	Route #	Dose Range
Aripiprazole	Abilify®, Abilify Discmelt® (ODT)	T, ODT, SI, SO	PO, IM	PO: 2-30 mg/day IM (immediate release injection): 9.75 mg as a single dose
Aripiprazole	Abilify Maintena®	SI (LAI)	IM	300-400 mg monthly
Aripiprazole lauroxil	Aristada®	SI (LAI)	IM	441-882 mg monthly
Asenapine	Saphris®	T	SL	2.5-10 mg BID
Brexpiprazole	Rexulti®	T	PO	0.25-4 mg/day
Cariprazine	Vraylar®	C	PO	1.5-6 mg/day
Clozapine	Clozaril®, FazaClo®, Versacloz®	T, ODT, SO	PO	12.5-900 mg/day
Iloperidone	Fanapt®	T	PO	1-12 mg BID
Lurasidone	Latuda®	T	PO	20-160 mg/day
Olanzapine	Zyprexa®, Zyprexa Zydis®, Zyprexa IM®	T, ODT, SI	PO, IM	PO: 2.5-20mg/day IM (immediate release injection): 10 mg as a single dose
Olanzapine	Zyprexa Relprevv™	SI (LAI)	IM	150-300 mg Q2WKs or 405 mg monthly
Paliperidone	Invega®	ERT	PO	3-12 mg/day
Paliperidone Palmitate	Invega Sustenna®	SI (LAI)	IM	39-234 mg monthly
Paliperidone Palmitate	Invega Trinza®	SI (LAI)	IM	273-819 mg every 3 months
Pimavanserin	Nuplazid™	T	PO	34 mg/day
Quetiapine	Seroquel®, Seroquel XR®	T, ERT	PO	25-800 mg/day
Risperidone	Risperdal®, Risperdal M-Tab®	T, SO, ODT	PO	0.25-16 mg/day
Risperidone	Risperdal Consta®	SI (LAI)	IM	12.5-50 mg q2 WKs
Ziprasidone	Geodon®	C, SI (mesylate)	PO, IM	PO: 20-80 mg BID IM: 10-40 mg/dose

*C: Capsule, ERT: Extended-Release Tablet, ODT: Orally Disintegrating Tablet, SI: Solution for Injection, T: Tablet, LAI: Long-Acting Injectable, SI: Solution/Suspension for Injection, SO: Solution for Oral Use. # PO: oral route, IM: intramuscularly, SL: Sublingual

45

Table 6 describes various pharmacokinetic profiles of atypical antipsychotics (second generation antipsychotics) including mechanism of action (MOA), half-life ($T_{1/2}$), and metabolizing/inhibited enzymes:[23-42]

Drug	MOA[#]	$T_{1/2}$ (Hours)*	Metabolism ^	Enzyme Inhibited^
Aripiprazole	Partial agonist at D_2 and $5HT_{1A}$	75, *94*	CYPs 2D6, 3A4	N/A
Asenapine[H]	D_2 and $5HT_{2A}$ antagonist	24	CYPs 1A2, 2D6, 3A4, UGT1A4	Weak CYP2D6
Brex-piprazole[H, R]	Partial agonist at D_2, D_3, and $5HT_{1A}$, antagonist at $5HT_{2A}$	91, *86*	CYPs 3A4, 2D6	N/A
Caripra-zine[H, R]	Partial agonist at D_2, and $5HT_{1A}$, antagonist at $5HT_{2A}$	2-4 days, *1-3 weeks*	CYPs 3A4, 2D6	Weak CYPs 1A2, 2C9, 2D6, 3A4, 2C19, 2A6, 2E1
Clozapine[H, R]	D_2 and $5HT_{2A}$ antagonist	12 hours	CYPs 1A2, 2D6, 3A4	CYPs 1A2, 2C9, 2E1
Iloperidone[H]	D_2 and $5HT_2$ antagonist	EM: 18, *26, 23* PM: 33, *37, 31*	P-gp, CYPs 2D6, 3A4	CYP3A4
Lurasidone[H, R]	D_2 and $5HT_{2A}$ antagonist, partial agonist at $5HT_{1A}$	18	CYP3A4	CYP3A4
Olanzapine[H]	$5HT_{2A}$, $5HT_{2C}$, D_{1-4}, H_1, α_1 antagonist	21-54, average: 30	CYPs 1A2, 2D6	CYPs 1A2, 2C9
Paliper-idone[R]	D_2 and $5HT_{2A}$ antagonist	23	P-gp, CYPs 2D6, 3A4	P-gp
Pimavan-serin[H, R]	Inverse agonist and antagonist at $5HT_{2A}$, $5HT_{2C}$, and sigma 1 receptors	57, *200*	CYPs 3A4, 3A5, 2J2, 2D6	N/A
Quetiapine[H]	D_2 and $5HT_2$ antagonist	IR: 6 ER: 7	CYP3A4	N/A
Risper-idone[H, R]	$5HT_2$, D_2 antagonist	EM: 3, *21* PM: 20, *30*	CYPs 2D6, 3A4	Weak CYP2D6
Ziprasidone[R]	D_2, $5HT_{2A}$, and $5HT_{1D}$, antagonist, $5HT_{1A}$ agonist	7	CYPs 3A4, 1A2, glutathione	N/A

[H]Caution advised in hepatic impairment   [R]Caution advised in renal impairment
*After Oral Administration, EM: Extensive Metabolizers, PM: Poor Metabolizers, *half-life of metabolites italicized.* ^CYP: Cytochrome, P-gp: P-glycoprotein.

Table 7 describes FDA approved indications for atypical antipsychotic drugs: [23-39, 42]

Drugs	Schizo-phrenia	Bipolar Disorder	MDD*, Adjunct	Others
Aripiprazole	X	X	X	Agitation, autistic irritability, mania, Tourette's
Asenapine	X	X		Mania
Brexpiprazole	X		X	
Cariprazine	X	X		Mania
Clozapine	X[Ψ]			Reduce Risk of Suicide Behavior[Φ]
Iloperidone	X			
Lurasidone	X	X		
Olanzapine	X	X		Agitation, mania, depression (with fluoxetine)
Paliperidone	X			Schizoaffective disorder
Pimavanserin				Parkinson's Disease Psychosis
Quetiapine	X	X	X (ER)	
Risperidone	X	X		Autistic Irritability
Ziprasidone	X	X		Agitation

[Ψ]: Treatment-refractory Schizophrenia; [Φ]: Reduction in Risk of Recurrent Suicidal Behavior in Schizophrenia or Schizoaffective Disorder; *MDD: Major Depressive Disorder.

Chlorpromazine (Thorazine®) [3, 43]
Available: 25 mg/mL (1 mL), 50 mg/2 mL (2 mL) solution for injection; 10, 25, 50, 100, 200 mg tablets.
Dose: **Schizophrenia, bipolar disorder, psychotic disorders:** *PO: Mild to moderate symptoms-* Initially 10 mg PO 3-4 times a day, or 25 mg PO 2-3 times per day. *Severe symptoms-* Initially 25 mg PO TID. After 1 or 2 days, may increase by 20-50 mg semi-weekly until symptoms controlled. Usual dose range 200-800 mg daily in 2-4 divided doses. **IM:** Initially 25 mg, may repeat 25-50 mg in one hour, gradually increase to max of 400 mg/dose every 4-6 hours. Usual dose 200-800 mg daily.
Intractable hiccups: *PO:* 25-50 mg PO 3-4 times a day. *IM (if no response to 2-3 days of PO therapy):* 25-50 mg as a single dose. *IV (if symptoms persist after PO and IM therapy):* 25-50 mg via slow IV infusion in 500-1000 mL of 0.9% Sodium Chloride for injection. Do not exceed IV rate of 1 mg/minute. *Monitor blood pressure closely, patient to remain flat in bed during entire infusion.*

Nausea/vomiting: *PO:* 10-25 mg PO every 4-6 hours PRN. *IM:* initially 12.5-25 mg, may repeat 25-50 mg IM every 3-4 hours PRN. Max: 1000 mg/day PO, up to 2000 mg for short periods.

<u>Renal:</u> Dosage adjustments not available per manufacturer's package insert. Use with caution. Not dialyzable.

<u>Hepatic:</u> Dosage adjustments not available per manufacturer's package insert. Use with caution.

- Injectable preparation contains sulfites- do not use in patients with sulfite hypersensitivity.
- Contraindicated in patients in comatose state.
- Contraindicated in patients receiving large amounts of CNS depressants (alcohol, barbiturates, narcotics, etc.)
- Skin hyperpigmentation (darkening of skin to slate gray color) may occur in rare instances in areas of body exposed to sunlight (primarily occurs in females who have received for 3+ years in dosages ranging from 500-1500mg/day)
- Ocular changes-occur more frequently than skin pigmentation (usually occur in patients receiving for 2+ years in dosages of 300mg/day and higher) characterized by deposition of fine particulate matter in lens and cornea.

<u>Droperidol (Inapsine®)</u> [4]

Available: 2.5 mg/mL (2 mL) solution for injection.

<u>Dose:</u> **Postoperative nausea/vomiting (PONV):** *IV/IM:* Maximum initial dose- 2.5 mg. Additional doses of 1.25 mg may be administered.

<u>Renal:</u> Dosage adjustments not available per manufacturer's package insert. Use with caution.

<u>Hepatic:</u> Dosage adjustments not available per manufacturer's package insert. Use with caution.

<u>Contraindicated</u> with known or suspected QT prolongation

<u>Fluphenazine (Prolixin®)</u> [5,6,7,44]

Available: 5 mg/mL (120 mL) oral concentrate; 2.5 mg/5 mL (60 mL, 473 mL) oral elixir; 25 mg/mL (5 mL) solution for injection as decanoate; 2.5 mg/mL (10 mL) Solution for injection as hydrochloride; 1, 2.5, 5, 10 mg Tablets.

<u>Dose:</u> **Schizophrenia:** *PO:* 2.5-10 mg PO in 2-3 divided doses. Max: 40 mg/day *IM/Subcutaneous (decanoate):* 12.5-25 mg every 3-4 weeks, may last up to 6 weeks. Increase in 12.5 mg increments. Max: 100 mg. *IM fluphenazine 12.5 mg decanoate every 3 weeks is approximately equivalent to 10 mg of oral HCl per day.* **Psychosis:** *IM (hydrochloride):* initially administer 1.25 mg as a single dose. May need 2.5-10 mg/day in divided dose at 6-8 hour interval. *IM fluphenazine HCl is approximately equivalent to 33% to 50% of oral fluphenazine HCl dose. Caution in paraben allergy.*

<u>Renal:</u> Dosage adjustments not available per manufacturer's package insert.

Hepatic: *Contraindicated* in patients with hepatic impairment. Depot injection formulation (decanoate) is contraindicated in patients with hepatic impairment.
- Contraindicated in patients with hematological disease.
- Fluphenazine hydrochloride is immediate release formulation. Fluphenazine decanoate is long-acting formulation. Intravenous administration of all fluphenazine injections should be avoided.
- Contraindicated for use in patients in comatose state.

Haloperidol (Haldol®) [8-10, 44-45]

Available: 2 mg/mL (5 mL, 15 mL, 120 mL) oral concentrate; 50 mg/mL (1 mL, 5 mL), 100 mg/mL (1 mL, 5 mL) solution as decanoate; 5 mg/mL (1 mL), 5 mg/mL (1 mL, 10 mL) solution as lactate; 0.5, 1, 2, 5, 10, 20 mg tablets.

Dose: **Schizophrenia:** *PO:* 0.5-2 mg PO 2-3 times per day. Usual dose range 5-20 mg/day. Doses up 100 mg/day may be necessary. *IM (as lactate):* 2-5 mg, subsequent doses may be given as often as 60 min. Given every 4-8 hours may be adequate. Max 20 mg/day. *IM (as decanoate):* initially, 10-20 times the oral dose. Initial dose should not exceed 100 mg. If initial dose conversion requires more than 100 mg, administer the dose in 2 injections separated by 3-7 days. For maintenance, provide 10-15 times the previous daily oral dose or 50 - 200 mg administered every 4 week interval. **Tourette syndrome:** *PO:* Initially, 0.5-2 mg PO 2-3 times per day. May increase to 3-5 mg PO 2-3 times per day. Average dose 15 mg/day. Max 100 mg/day.

Renal: Dosage adjustments not available per manufacturer's package insert.
Hepatic: Dosage adjustments not available per manufacturer's package insert. Use with caution. Haloperidol extensively metabolized in the liver.
- Haloperidol decanoate is for intramuscular use only, must not be administered intravenously.
- Haloperidol lactate is not FDA approved for intravenous administration if given IV should be monitored via EKG for QT prolongation.
- Haloperidol is contraindicated in patients who are in a coma or who exhibit severe toxic CNS depression.
- Some oral formulations of haloperidol may contain tartrazine dye or other yellow dyes.

Molindone (Moban®) [11]

Available: 5, 10, 25, 50 mg tablets.

Dose: **Schizophrenia:** Initial: 50-75 mg/day divided in 3-4 doses, may increase to 100 mg/day in 3-4 days. Max 225 mg/day. Maintenance: 5-15 mg for mild symptoms, or 10-25 mg for moderate symptoms given 3-4 times/day. Up to 225 mg/day may be required for severe symptoms. Max 225 mg/day PO.
Renal: Dosage adjustments not available per manufacturer's package insert.
Hepatic: Dosage adjustments not available per manufacturer's package insert. Use with caution.

Perphenazine (Trilafon®) [12]

Available: 2, 4, 8, 16 mg tablets.

Dose: **Schizophrenia:** 4-8 mg PO TID. Max 24 mg/day. 8-16 mg PO 2-3 times per day (max 64 mg/day) in hospitalized patients.

Severe nausea/vomiting: 8-16 mg/day in divided doses. Max 24 mg/day.

Renal: Dosage adjustments not available per manufacturer's package insert.

Hepatic: *Contraindicated* in patients with significant hepatic impairment.

Pimozide (Orap®) [13]

Available: 1, 2 mg tablets.

Dose: **Tourette disorder:** initially 1-2 mg/day in divided doses. Then increase dose as needed every other day. Max 10 mg/day, or 0.2 mg/kg/day, whichever is less.

Renal: Dosage adjustments not available per manufacturer's package insert. Use with caution, as metabolites are excreted primarily through the kidney.

Hepatic: Dosage adjustments not available per manufacturer's package insert. However, pimozide is extensively metabolized by dealkylation in the liver. Use with caution.

- CYP2D6 genotyping recommended, given metabolism of pimozide by CYP2D6 and the potential for toxicity. For those that are CYP2D6 poor metabolizers, dose increase should occur no earlier than 14 days, and max daily dose should not exceed 4 mg/day.
- Contraindicated with potent CYP2D6 or CYP3A4 inhibitors due to potential for QT prolongation or Torsade de Pointes (TdP.)
- Contraindicated in patients with simple tics or other tics which are unrelated to Tourette's syndrome.
- Pimozide is contraindicated during use of other drugs known to cause tics, such as pemoline, methylphenidate, and amphetamines, until these drugs are excluded as a potential cause of the tics.

Prochlorperazine (Compazine®; Compro®) [14,15]

Available: 5 mg/mL (2 mL) solution for injection; 25 mg rectal suppository; 5, 10 mg tablets.

Dose: **Schizophrenia:** 5-10mg 3-4 times per day. **Nausea/vomiting:** *PO:* 5-10 mg PO 3-4 times per day. Max 40 mg/day. *Rectal:* 25 mg per rectum BID. *IM (as edisylate):* 5-10 mg every 3-4 hours, max 40 mg/day. *IV (as edisylate):* 2.5-10 mg; max 10 mg/dose. IV infusion rate not to exceed 5 mg per minute. May repeat every 3-4 hours as needed. Max 40 mg/day.

Renal: Dosage adjustments not available per manufacturer's package insert.

Hepatic: Dosage adjustments not available per manufacturer's package insert. Use with caution, as drug undergoes hepatic metabolism.

Thioridazine (Mellaril®) [16]

Available: 10, 25, 50, 100 mg tablets.

Dose: **Schizophrenia:** Initially 50-100 mg PO TID. Titrate to total daily dose of 200-800 mg/day.

Renal: Dosage adjustments not available per manufacturer's package insert. Not removed by hemodialysis.

Hepatic: Dosage adjustments not available per manufacturer's package insert. Use with caution, as drug undergoes hepatic metabolism.

- Contraindicated with potent CYP2D6 inhibitors due to potential for QT prolongation or Torsade de Pointes (TdP.)

Thiothixene (Navane®) [17]

Available: 1, 2, 5, 10 mg capsules.

Dose: **Schizophrenia:** Mild-to-moderate symptoms: 2 mg PO TID, usual dose 15 mg/day. Severe symptoms: 5 mg BID, usual dose 20-30 mg/day. Increase gradually. Max 60 mg/day.

Renal: Dosage adjustments not available per manufacturer's package insert.

Hepatic: Dosage adjustments not available per manufacturer's package insert. Patients who develop jaundice secondary to thiothixene use should have therapy discontinued.

- Patients with hypocalcemia may be at an increased risk for having dystonic reactions, use with caution.

Trifluoperazine (Stelazine®) [18]

Available: 1, 2, 5, 10 mg tablets.

Dose: **Schizophrenia:** initially 2-5 mg PO BID. Titrate gradually based on response and tolerability. Usual dose 15-20 mg/day in divided doses. Some may require 40 mg/day. **Nonpsychotic anxiety:** 1-2 mg PO BID. Max 6 mg/day. Do not exceed doses of more than 6 mg per day for longer than 12 weeks due to risk for tardive dyskinesia.

Renal: Dosage adjustments not available per manufacturer's package insert.

Hepatic: Dosage adjustments not available per manufacturer's package insert. Use contraindicated in patients with hepatic disease.

Second Generation Antipsychotics (SGAs) [23-25, 49, 26-28, 52, 29-38, 55]

- **FDA Black Box Warning (BBW) regarding all SGAs in treatment of dementia-related psychosis in elderly:**
  In April 2005 the FDA mandated that all manufacturers of atypical antipsychotics include a boxed warning to the labeling indicating that increased death rates (1.6—1.7 times that of placebo) have been noted in this patient population receiving atypical antipsychotics. Death typically occurred due to heart failure, sudden death, or infections (primarily pneumonia).[46]
- **DRESS (Drug Reaction with Eosinophilia and Systemic Symptoms) has been reported with the following:**
  Olanzapine, Quetiapine, Ziprasidone.[47]
- **Caution in conditions (bradycardia, hypokalemia/hypomagnesemia, presence of congenital prolongation of QT interval, recent acute myocardial infarct, uncompensated heart failure) or when combined with drugs that may prolong QT interval as this may result in torsades de pointes and/or sudden death.** [58-61]
- **FDA approved a labeling update for ALL antipsychotic medications adding new warning that antipsychotics can cause somnolence, postural hypotension and motor instability that could lead to falls and subsequently fractures or other injuries.**

MOA: Blockade of $5HT_2$ and dopamine antagonism. There are many different receptors that the various SGAs have antagonist/amongst partial agonist activities (i.e. histamine H_1, $alpha_{1/2A/2C}$, dopamine (D_{1-5})), muscarinic (M_{1-5}) and serotonin ($5HT_{1A-D/2A-C/3/5/6/7}$). The varying antagonism may help to explain the countless side effects from each individual drug.

Adverse Effects: As noted above varies from individual drug. Some common ones are akathisia, dizziness, drowsiness, EPS, insomnia, metabolic dysfunction, orthostatic hypotension, QT prolongation, weight gain, etc.

Contraindications: Intolerance/allergic reaction to particular compound. See individual drug for contraindications.

Metabolic monitoring parameters per ADA & APA consensus guidelines [48]:

	Baseline	Week 4	Week 8	Quarterly	Annually
Medical History[1]	X			X	X
Weight (BMI)	X	X	X	X	X
Waist circumference	X			X	X
Blood pressure	X			X	X
Fasting glucose	X			X	X
Fasting lipids	X			X	X

[1]Personal & family history of obesity, diabetes, hypertension and cardiovascular disease

Dose Comparison of Atypical Antipsychotics in Children & Adolescents:

	Schizo-phrenia	Bipolar I disorder	Autistic Disorder	Usual dose (mg/day)	Max dose (mg/day)
Aripiprazole	13-17 years	10-17 years	6-17 years	2 – 10	30
Asenapine		10-17 years			
Lurasidone	13-17 years			40 – 80	80
Olanzapine	13-17 years	13-17 years		2.5 – 10	20
Paliperidone	12-17 years				
Quetiapine	13-17 years	10-17 years		50 – 400	800
Risperidone	13-17 years	10-17 years	5-16 years	0.5 – 3	6

Aripiprazole (Abilify®/DISCMELT®/Maintena®/Aristada®) [49-51, 23-25]
Available: 1 mg/mL oral solution; 10 and 15 mg oral disintegrating tablets; 2, 5, 10, 15, 20 and 30 mg tablets; 300 and 400 mg extended-release powder for injection or pre-filled dual chamber syringe for injection; 441 mg/1.6mL, 662mg/2.4 mL and 882 mg/3.2mL extended-release suspension for injection

Dose: SEE *LAI TABLE* FOR LAI INJECTION DOSING
Schizophrenia: 10-15 mg daily may increase to dose of 30 mg/day.
MDD, adjunct: 2-5 mg daily may gradually increase up to 15 mg daily.
Bipolar: 15 mg daily (monotherapy) or 10-15 mg daily (adjunctive) may increase upward to 30 mg daily. Max dose 30 mg/day tablets; 25 mg/day oral solution; 400 mg/month extended release IM (Maintena®); 882 mg /month extended release IM (Aristada®).
Renal: No adjustment
Hepatic: No adjustment

- Long half-life of ~75 hours; therefore, steady state (SS) attained ~14 days after oral dose. Caution with rapid dose escalation as delayed SS.
- Reduced dosing necessary with CYP2D6 & CYP3A4 inhibitors or poor metabolizers as below
- Oral solution can be substituted on mg-per-mg basis for tablet up to 25 mg solution (30 mg tablets should receive 25 mg of solution due to enhanced absorption of solution at higher doses)
- Aristada® is a pro-drug of Aripiprazole-after IM administration conversion via enzyme-mediated hydrolysis & then water-mediated hydrolysis occurs
- See LAI table for details on Maintena® (PO overlap x 14 days & SS at 4th dose) and Aristada® (PO overlap x 21 days)

- Watch for compulsive behaviors, akathisia, insomnia, nausea/vomiting, headache and anxiety
- Rare events of QT prolongation have occurred

Dose Adjustment Chart:

FACTORS	DOSE ADJUSTMENTS
Known CYP2D6 Poor Metabolizers	Administer ½ usual dose
Known CYP2D6 Poor Metabolizers + Strong CYP3A4 Inhibitors	Administer ¼ usual dose
Strong CYP2D6 **OR** 3A4 Inhibitors	Administer ½ usual dose
Strong CYP2D6 **AND** 3A4 Inhibitor	Administer ¼ usual dose
Strong CYP3A4 Inducer	Double usual dose over 1-2 weeks

Aristada® Doses Based Upon Oral Aripiprazole Total Daily Dose:

Aripiprazole (PO)	Aripiprazole (PO)	Aristada®
10mg/day	300mg/month	441mg/month
15mg/day	450mg/month	662mg/month
≥20mg/day	600mg/month	882mg/month

Maintena® Approximate Dose Equivalency Upon Oral Aripiprazole Total Daily Dose:

Aripiprazole (PO)	Abilify Maintena®
16mg/day	300mg/month
21mg/day	400mg/month

Asenapine (Saphris®) [26]

Available: 2.5, 5 and 10 mg sublingual tablets

Dose: **Schizophrenia:** 5 mg BID; may increase to 10 mg BID. **Bipolar:** 5-10mg BID. Max dose 20 mg/day.

Renal: No adjustment

Hepatic: *Severe impairment*—not recommended (exposure 7 times higher)

- Drinking water 2-5 minutes after administration (decreases exposure 19% and 10% respectively)
- **DO NOT EAT OR DRINK FOR 10 MINUTES AFTER ADMINISTRATION**
- **Reduce dose by ½ with CYP2D6 Inhibitors**
- Watch for akathisia, constipation, drowsiness, hyperglycemia, hypertriglyceridemia and weight gain
- Serious allergic reactions and angioedema have been reported
- Has not exhibited significant QT prolongation (~2-5 msec compared to placebo; cardiac precautions remain for all antipsychotics)

Brexpiprazole (Rexulti®) [27]

Available: 0.25, 0.5, 1, 2, 3 and 4 mg tablets

Dose: **Schizophrenia:** 1 mg daily x 4 days, then 2 mg daily x 3 days, then 4 mg daily based upon response and tolerability. Max dose 4 mg/day. **MDD, adjunct**: 0.5-1 mg daily; may increase to 1 mg then 2 mg daily in weekly intervals based upon response/tolerance. Max dose 3 mg/day.

Renal: *CrCl < 60mL/min (including ESRD):* max dose of 2 mg/day for MDD and 3 mg/day for schizophrenia.

Hepatic: *Moderate to severe impairment (Child-Pugh ≥ 7)* max dose of 2 mg/day for MDD and 3 mg/day for schizophrenia.

- Reduced dosing necessary with CPY2D6 & CYP3A4 inhibitors or poor metabolizers as below.
- Watch for dyspepsia, headache, constipation and akathisia.
- At 4 times the maximum human recommended dose--did not prolong QTc interval to clinically relevant extent.

Dose Adjustment Chart:

FACTORS	DOSE ADJUSTMENTS
Strong CYP2D6* **OR** 3A4 Inhibitors	Administer ½ usual dose
Known CYP2D6 Poor Metabolizers + Strong/moderate CYP3A4 Inhibitors	Administer ¼ usual dose
Strong/moderate CYP2D6 **AND** Strong/moderate 3A4 Inhibitor	Administer ¼ usual dose
Strong CYP3A4 Inducer	Double usual dose and further adjust based upon clinical response

May be administered without dose adjustment in patients with MDD when administered with strong CYP2D6 inhibitors (i.e. paroxetine, fluoxetine)

Cariprazine (Vraylar®) [52]

Available: 1.5, 3, 4.5, 6 mg capsules

Dose: **Schizophrenia/Bipolar:** 1.5 mg daily on day 1 increased to 3 mg daily. Further adjustments can be made in 1.5-3 mg increments based upon response/tolerability. Max dose: 6 mg/day.

Renal: *Severe impairment (CrCl < 30ml/min):* not recommended.

Hepatic: *Severe impairment (Child-Pugh 10-15):* not recommended.

- Long half-life; dose changes will not reflect for several weeks.
- **Strong CYP3A4 Inhibitors: reduce dose by half.**
- Watch for EPS, akathisia and somnolence.
- At doses 3 times human maximum recommended dose—did not prolong QTc interval to clinically relevant extent.

Clozapine (Clozaril®; FazaClo®; VERSACLOZ®) [28, 53-54]

Available: 25, 50, 100 and 200 mg tablets; 12.5, 25, 100, 150 and 200 mg oral disintegrating tablets; 50 mg/1 mL oral suspension

Dose: 12.5 mg daily or BID then slowly titrated in increments of 25-50 mg/day to target dose of 300-450 mg/day in divided doses by end of 2 weeks. Max dose 900 mg/day.

Renal: May need to *reduce* dose in significant renal impairment

Hepatic: *Modify* dose depending upon clinical response & degree of impairment. If signs/symptoms of liver impairment, LFTs should be measured, if significantly elevated or jaundice present-treatment should be discontinued

- Risk of severe neutropenia—ALL patients must be enrolled in Clozapine REMS Program—www.clozapinerems.com or 1-844-267-8678
- Indicated/reserved for treatment-resistant schizophrenia & reducing suicidal behavior in patients with schizophrenia
- Black Box Warning: Bradycardia, Cardiomyopathy, Dementia, Myocarditis, Neutropenia, Orthostatic Hypotension, Seizures and Syncope and contraindicated in agranulocytosis, coma and ileus.
- Risk of orthostatic hypotension/bradycardia/syncope is highest during initial titration period (particularly with rapid dose escalation) and seizures risks appear to be dose-related. Additionally watch for dizziness, sedation, weight gain, hyperglycemia and constipation
- Reduce dose by one-third when coadministered with Strong CYP1A2 Inhibitors
- Concomitant use of Strong CYP3A4 Inducers is not recommended and may be necessary to reduce dose with CYP2D6 inhibitors or poor metabolizers
- Re-initiation should occur if 2 days or more have elapsed since last dose.
- Gradual dose reduction over 1-2 weeks is recommended in discontinuation unless clinical circumstances (i.e. neutropenia) require abrupt discontinuation with continued ANC monitoring for 2 weeks post discontinuation
- Caution when administered with other drugs that may prolong QT interval
- Smoking (hydrocarbons—not nicotine) will reduce Clozapine levels via CYP1A2 induction.

A Recommended Clozapine Dosage Titration at Start of Therapy (*Optional)

Week 1	AM (mg)	HS (mg)	Total (mg)	Week 2	AM (mg)	HS (mg)	Total (mg)
Day 1	12.5	12.5*	12.5-25	Day 8	50	100	150
Day 2	25	---	25	Day 9	100	100	200
Day 3	25	25	50	Day 10	100	100	200
Day 4	25	50	75	Day 11	50	200	250
Day 5	50	50	100	Day 12	50	200	250
Day 6	50	75	125	Day 13	100	200	300
Day 7	50	100	150	Day 14	100	200	300

Clozapine Treatment Monitoring
For General Population & Benign Ethnic Neutropenia (BEN) [62]

ANC LEVEL	Clozapine Treatment Recommendations	ANC Monitoring
Normal Range (≥ 1500/µL) BEN Population: ANC ≥ 1000/µL**	Initiate treatment. If treatment interrupted: - < 30 days continue monitoring as before - ≥ 30 days, monitor as if new patient	Weekly from initiation to 6 months → Every 2 weeks from 6-12 months → Monthly after 12 months
Mild Neutropenia (1000-1499/µL)*	Continue treatment	Three times weekly until ANC ≥ 1500/uL. Once ANC ≥ 1500/uL return to patient's last "Normal Range" ANC monitoring interval.
	BEN Population: Mild neutropenia is normal range for BEN population.** Continue treatment as outlined under Normal Range.	*BEN Population:* Weekly from initiation to 6 months → Every 2 weeks from 6-12 months → Monthly after 12 months
Moderate Neutropenia (500-999/µL)*	Recommend hematology consult. Interrupt treatment for suspected clozapine-induced neutropenia. Resume treatment once ANC ≥ 1000/µL.	Daily until ANC ≥ 1000/uL then three times weekly until ANC ≥ 1500/uL. Once ANC ≥ 1500/uL check ANC weekly for 4 weeks then return to patient's last "Normal Range" ANC monitoring interval.
	BEN Population: Recommend hematology consult. Continue treatment.	*BEN Population:* Three times weekly until ANC ≥ 1000/µL or ≥ patient's known baseline Once ANC ≥ 1000/µL or at patient's known baseline, check ANC weekly for 4 weeks, then return to patient's last "Normal BEN Range" ANC monitoring interval
Severe Neutropenia (< 500/µL)*	General & BEN Population: Recommend hematology consult. Interrupt treatment for suspected clozapine-induced neutropenia. Do not rechallenge unless prescriber determines benefits outweigh risks.	Daily until ANC ≥ 1000/µL then three times weekly until ANC ≥ 1500/µL. If patient rechallenged, resume treatment as new patient.
		BEN Population: Daily until ANC ≥ 500/µL then three times weekly until ANC ≥ patient's baseline. If patient rechallenged, resume treatment as new patient once ANC ≥1000/µL or at baseline.

*Confirm all initial reports of ANC < 1500/uL with a repeat ANC measurement within 24 hours. **Obtain at least 2 baseline ANC levels before initiating treatment.*

Iloperidone (Fanapt®) [29]

Available: 1, 2, 4, 6, 8, 10 and 12 mg tablets

Dose: **Schizophrenia:** 1 mg BID initially; may increase by up to 2 mg BID to target dose of 6-12 mg BID. Max dose 24 mg/day.

Renal: No adjustment

Hepatic: *Moderate:* use caution; *Severe:* not recommended

- Reduce dose by half with CYP2D6 & CYP 3A4 inhibitors or poor metabolizers
- Watch for dizziness, orthostatic hypotension and somnolence
- If stopped for more than 3 days, requires dose re-titration.
- QT_c prolongation of 9 msec at 12 mg BID & ~19 msec at 12 mg BID with 2D6 or 3A4 inhibitor

Lurasidone (Latuda®) [30]

Available: 20, 40, 60, 80 and 120 mg tablets

Dose: **Schizophrenia:** 40 mg daily; may increase to max dose of 160 mg/day. **Bipolar:** 20 mg daily; may increase to max dose of 120 mg/day.

Renal: *CrCl < 50 mL/min:* initial dose of 20mg/day with max of 80 mg/day

Hepatic: *Moderate impairment (Child Pugh 7-9):* initial dose of 20 mg/day with max of 80 mg/day. *Severe impairment (Child Pugh 10-15):* initial dose of 20 mg/day with max of 40 mg/day

- Administer with food (at least 350 calories)
- Watch for nausea, somnolence and dose-related akathisia
- Dose adjust for moderate CYP 3A4 inhibitors
- **Not recommended in strong CYP 3A4 inhibitors or inducers**
- Maximum mean (upper 1-sided, 95% CI) increase in baseline-adjusted QTc intervals based on individual correction method (QTcI) was 7.5 (11.7) msec for 120mg.

Olanzapine (Zyprexa®; Relprevv™; Zydis®) [31]

Available: 2.5, 5, 7.5, 10, 15 and 20 mg tablets; 5, 10, 15 and 20 mg oral disintegrating tablets; 10 mg powder for solution for injection; 210, 300 and 405 mg (extended release) powder for suspension for injection

Dose: **SEE *LAI TABLE* FOR LAI INJECTION DOSING**

Schizophrenia: 5-10 mg with further dose adjustments by 5 mg/day if indicated at weekly intervals. Max dose 20 mg/day. **Bipolar:** 10-15 mg daily with further dose adjustments by 5 mg/day if indicated but no less than 24 hours apart. Max dose 20 mg/day. **Agitation:** 10 mg IM x 1 dose; may repeat in 2 hours and then again 4 hours after 2nd dose. Max dose 30 mg/day of immediate-release IM.

Max Dose for extended release IM: 300 mg every 2 Weeks or 405 mg every 4 Weeks (see table below for dosing on olanzapine extended release IM).

Renal: No adjustment

<u>Hepatic:</u> Use *lower* starting doses with careful titration based upon degree of impairment and clinical response

- If at risk for hypotension initiate at lower dose
- Watch for sedation, weight gain, hyperglycemia, hypertriglyceridemia, hypercholesterolemia and constipation
- No significant changes in QT interval; however, there have been case reports of QT prolongation
- Black box warning (BBW) of post-injection delirium/sedation syndrome (PDSS) in Relprevv™
- Clearance 40% higher in smokers (CYP1A2 induction) than nonsmokers
- REMS program for https://www.zyprexarelprevvprogram.com

Recommended Dosing for Zyprexa Relprevv™ from Oral Zyprexa® Doses

Zyprexa® Oral Dose	Zyprexa Relprevv™ During 1st 8 Weeks	Zyprexa Relprevv™ After 8 Weeks (Maintenance Dose)
10 mg/day	210 mg/Q2 Weeks OR 405 mg/Q4 Weeks	150 mg/Q2 Weeks OR 300 mg/Q4 Weeks
15 mg/day	300 mg/Q2 Weeks	210 mg/Q2 Weeks OR 405 mg/Q4 Weeks
20 mg/day	300 mg Q2 Weeks	300 mg Q2 Weeks

<u>Paliperidone (Invega®/Sustenna®/Trinza®)</u> [32-34]

Available: 1.5, 3, 6 and 9 mg extended-release tablets; 39, 78, 117, 156 and 234 mg extended-release suspension for monthly injection (Sustenna®); 273, 410, 546 and 819 mg extended-release suspension for every 3-month injection (Trinza®)

<u>Dose:</u> **SEE *LAI TABLE* FOR LAI INJECTION DOSING**

Schizophrenia/SCAD: 6 mg QAM (lower dose of 3 mg/day may be sufficient); may increase by 3 mg/day every 5 days up to max dose of 12 mg/day.

Max Dose: Sustenna® -234 mg every 4 weeks & Trinza®-819 mg every 3 Months.

<u>Renal:</u> **PO:** *CrCl 50-79 mL/min:* initial 3 mg/day with max of 6 mg/day; CrCl 10-49 mL/min: initial 1.5 mg/day and max of 3 mg/day; *CrCl < 10mL/min:* not recommended. **IM (Sustenna®):** *CrCl 50-79 mL/min:* Initiate 156 mg IM day 1; 117 mg 2nd dose a week later and 78 mg IM once monthly thereafter. **IM (Trinza®):** *CrCl 50-79 mL/min:* Only for patients stabilized on Invega Sustenna®—conversion based on previous stabilized dose of Sustenna®. *CrCl < 50mL/min:* not recommended in either IM formulation.

<u>Hepatic:</u> No adjustment

- Half-life: PO-23 hours, once-month depot-25-49 days; 3-month depot-84-95 days in deltoid & 118-139 days in gluteal.
- Watch for akathisia, hypercholesterolemia, hyperglycemia, hyperlipidemia, hyperprolactinemia/galactorrhea, orthostatic hypotension and constipation

- Modest increase in QTc interval (8 mg resulted in ~12.3 msec increase from baseline in QTcLD-interval corrected for heart rate using population specific linear derived method)

Approximate Dose Equivalencies:

Risperdal Consta®	Invega® Tablet (PO)	Invega Sustenna®	Invega Trinza®
25 mg Q2 Weeks	3 mg/day	78 mg Q4 Weeks	273 mg Q3 Month
37.5 mg Q2 Weeks	6 mg/day	117 mg Q4 Weeks	410 mg Q3 Month
50 mg Q2 Weeks	9 mg/day	156 mg Q4 Weeks	546 mg Q3 Month
	12 mg/day	234 mg Q4 Weeks	819 mg Q3 Month

Conversion from Invega Sustenna® 39mg was not studied.
Trinza® conversion dose is 3.5 times the Sustenna° dose.

Pimavanserin (Nuplazid™)[42]
Available: 17 mg tablets

Dose: **Parkinson disease psychosis:** 34 mg PO daily. Concomitant therapy with strong CYP3A4 inhibitors (eg, ketoconazole): 17 mg once daily.
Concomitant therapy with strong CYP3A4 inducers: 34 mg once daily; monitor for reduced efficacy, may need dosage increase.
Renal: *CrCl ≥30 mL/min:* no dosage adjustment necessary. *CrCl <30 mL/min:* use not recommended; not studied.
Hepatic: Use *not recommended*; not studied.

Quetiapine (Seroquel®/XR®) [35-36]
Available: 25, 50, 100, 200, 300 and 400 mg tablets; 50, 150, 200, 300 and 400 mg extended-release tablets

Dose: **Schizophrenia: IR tablets:** 25 mg BID Day 1; increase by 25-50 mg BID-TID Days 2 & 3 to target range of 300-400 mg/day in divided doses by Day 4. Further increments of 25-50 mg BID in intervals of no less than 2 days. **ER tablets:** 300 mg daily; may titrate in intervals of 300 mg/day. **Bipolar: IR tablets:** 50 mg BID Day 1; increase increments of up to 100 mg/day in divided doses to 400 mg/day on Day 4; may further increase up to 800 mg/day by Day 6. **ER tablets:** 300 mg daily Day 1 followed by 600 mg daily Day 2. May adjust dose day 3 based upon response/tolerance. Max Dose: 800 mg/day. **MDD, adjunct:** 50 mg daily on Day 1 & 2; 150 mg daily Day 3. Effectiveness has been demonstrated at range of 150-300 mg/day
Renal: No adjustment
Hepatic: Impairment *reduces* clearance by 30%. **IR tablets:** 25mg daily Day 1 & increase by 25-50 mg/day. **ER tablets:** 50 mg daily Day 1 & increase by 50 mg/day. Use lowest effective & tolerable dose.
- **Strong CYP3A4 Inhibitors: reduce dose to 1/6th dose**
- **Strong CYP3A4 Inducers: increase dose 5-fold**
- Re-titrate if therapy is discontinued for more than a week

- Watch for constipation, drowsiness, hypercholesterolemia, hypertriglyceridemia, orthostatic hypotension and weight gain
- Food (800-1000 calories) significantly increases Cmax & AUC of ER tablet Should be given without meal or light snack only (300 calories or less)
- Not associated with persistent increases in QT interval; however, case reports of QT prolongation so caution with other QT prolonging drugs

Risperidone (Risperdal®/M-Tab®/Consta®) [37-38, 55-56]

Available: 1 mg/mL oral solution; 0.25, 0.5, 1, 2, 3 and 4 mg tablets; 0.25, 0.5, 1, 2, 3 and 4 mg oral disintegrating tablets; 12.5, 25, 37.5 and 50 mg (extended release) powder for suspension for injection

Dose: SEE *LAI TABLE* FOR LAI INJECTION DOSING

Schizophrenia: 2 mg daily or 1 mg BID; may increase by 1-2 mg/day to target dose of 4-8 mg/day. Max Dose: 16 mg/day. **Bipolar:** 2-3 mg/day; may increase by 1 mg/day to max dose of 6 mg/day. Max Dose: 50 mg IM Q2 Weeks for Consta®

Renal: *CrCl < 30mL/min:* initiate 0.5 mg BID & titrate in increments of 0.5 mg/day or less. In doses of 1.5 mg BID titrate in weekly intervals.

Hepatic: *Severe impairment (Child Pugh 10-15):* initiate 0.5 mg BID & titrate in increments of 0.5 mg/day or less. Doses of 1.5 mg BID titrate in weekly intervals.

- Dose > 6 mg/day associated with more extrapyramidal side effects (EPS).
- PO overlap for 3 weeks after first Consta® depot injection.
- Reduce initial dose with CYP 2D6 Inhibitors; Do not exceed 8 mg/day.
- Watch for akathisia, constipation, hyperprolactinemia/galactorrhea, EPS, hypercholesterolemia, hyperlipidemia, hypertriglyceridemia and orthostatic hypotension.
- Not associated with persistent increases in QT interval; however, case reports of QT prolongation so caution with other QT prolonging drugs.

Approximate Dose Equivalencies:

Risperdal®	Risperdal Consta®
2 mg/day	25 mg Q2 Weeks
3 mg/day	37.5 mg Q2 Weeks
4 mg/day	50 mg Q2 Weeks

Ziprasidone (Geodon®) [39, 57]

Available: 20, 40, 60 and 80 mg capsules; 20 mg powder for injection

<u>Dose:</u> **Schizophrenia:** 20 mg BID; increase as needed at intervals of 2 days or more. Max Dose: 160 mg/day. **Bipolar:** 40 mg BID Day 1 may increase to 60-80 mg BID thereafter **Agitation***:* 10-20 mg IM per dose. Doses of 10mg IM may be given Q2H PRN & doses of 20 mg IM may be given every 4 hours PRN. Max Dose: 40 mg/day.

<u>Renal:</u> IM-use with *caution* due to cyclodextrin sodium excipient

<u>Hepatic:</u> No adjustment

- Do not use in combination with other drugs that have demonstrated QT prolongation. Discontinue in any patient with persistent QT interval > 500msec
- Contraindicated in acute myocardial infarction, heart failure, long QT syndrome and QT prolongation
- The mean increase in QT_c from baseline ranged from 9-14 msec more than (risperidone, olanzapine, quetiapine and haloperidol) but ~14 msec less than thioridazine.
- Watch for akathisia, insomnia, nausea/vomiting and headache
- Administer with food (500-1000 kcal) increases bioavailability by 2-fold.

LONG ACTING INJECTABLES (LAIs)[5-9, 24-25, 31, 33-34, 38, 50, 56]

	Generic name	Initial dose	Maintenance dose	~ Oral daily dose to IM conversion	Frequency	PO Overlap	Injection Site (IM)	Injection allowed since last dose
Haldol Decanoate®	Haloperidol decanoate*#	10-20x PO dose. Max 100 mg 1st injection. If >100mg give 100 mg then balance in 3-7 Days	Based on patient response	10-20x PO dose	4 weeks	No	Deltoid/ Gluteal	N/A
Prolixin Decanoate®	Fluphenazine decanoate*#	12.5mg-25mg	Based on patient response	PO = IM 1mg = 1.25mg	2-4 weeks	No	Deltoid/ Gluteal	N/A
Risperdal Consta®	Risperidone micros-phorox◊	25 mg	25-50 mg	PO = IM 2mg = 25mg 3mg = 37.5mg 4mg = 50mg	2 weeks	21 days	Deltoid/ Gluteal	± 3 days from next due date
Invega Sustenna®	Paliperidone palmitate◊¥	234mg Day 1 156mg 1 week later both in **Deltoid**	39-234mg	PO = IM 3mg = 39-78mg 6mg = 117mg 9mg = 156mg 12mg = 234mg	4 weeks	No	Deltoid/ Gluteal	Loading: 2nd dose ± 4 days from 1-week time point Maintenance: ± 7 from monthly due date
Invega Trinza®	paliperidone palmitate◊¥	Must be stable on Sustenna for ≥4months & last 2 doses same Sustenna--Trinza 78mg = 273mg 117mg = 410mg 156mg = 546mg 234mg = 819mg	Based on patient response	Not specified (3.5 X Sustenna Dose)	3 months	No	Deltoid/ Gluteal	Initial: ± 7 days from Sustenna dose due date Maintenance: ± 2 weeks from next Trinza dose
Abilify Maintena®	aripiprazole extended release◊†	400mg	300-400mg	PO = IM 16mg=300mg 21mg = 400mg	4 weeks	14 days	Deltoid/ Gluteal	≥ 26 days from last injection
Aristada®	aripiprazole lauroxil◊†	441mg 662mg 882mg	441mg, 662mg And 882mg	PO = IM 10mg = 441mg 15mg = 662mg 20mg = 882mg	4 weeks or 882 mg q6 weeks	21 days	Gluteal; 441mg may be Deltoid	≥ 14 days from last injection
Zyprexa Relprevv™	olanzapine pamoate◊∞	Table 1 Below	Table 1 Below	Table 1 Below	2-4 weeks	No	Gluteal	N/A

*-Caution in benzyl alcohol & sesame allergies   #Room Temp/Protect from light   ∞BBW-PDSS & REMS requirement   ◊Room Temp
◊-Refrigerate (room temp up to 7d-protect from light)   ¥-Renal impairment requires dosing adjustments
†-Coadministration with CYP2D6 & CYP3A4 Inhibitors requires dosing adjustments

Table 1-Recommended Dosing for Zyprexa Relprevv™

Zyprexa® Oral Dose	Zyprexa Relprevv™ During 1st 8 Weeks	Zyprexa Relprevv™ After 8 Weeks (Maintenance Dose)
10 mg/day	210 mg/Q2 Weeks OR 405 mg/Q4 Weeks	150 mg/Q2 Weeks OR 300mg/Q4 Weeks
15 mg/day	300 mg/Q2 Weeks	210 mg/Q2 Weeks OR 405 mg/Q4 Weeks
20 mg/day	300 mg Q2 Weeks	300 mg Q2 Weeks

Table 2-Invega Sustenna® 2nd Initiation Dose Missed

Week from 1st Injection	Instructions
< 4 Weeks	156mg ASAP & 117mg dose 5 weeks after 1st injection (regardless of timing of 2nd injection thereafter resume monthly dosing)
4-7 Weeks	156mg followed by 156mg 1 week later (both deltoid,) thereafter resume monthly dosing
>7 Weeks	Restart titration of 234mg then 156mg 1 week later (deltoid)

Table 3-Invega Sustenna® Maintenance Dose Missed

Time from Last Dose	Instructions
4 to 6 weeks	Resume usual monthly dose ASAP
>6 weeks to 6 months	Give 1 injection of usual monthly dose ASAP & another injection (same dose-both deltoid) 1 week later; thereafter, resume monthly dosing.*
>6 months	Restart titration of 234mg then 156mg 1 week later (deltoid)

Table 4-Abilify Maintena® Missed Dose

Dose was missed	Time since last injection	Instructions
2nd or 3rd dose	>4 weeks and < 5 weeks	Give injection ASAP
2nd or 3rd dose	>5 weeks	Restart concomitant oral aripiprazole for 14 days with next injection
4th or subsequent dose	>4 weeks and < 6 weeks	Give injection ASAP
4th or subsequent dose	>6 weeks	Restart concomitant oral aripiprazole for 14 days with next injection

Table 5 – Aristada® Missed Dose (Dose missed-administer next injection of Aristada® ASAP. Use PO supplementation as below)

Dose of Patient's Last Aristada® Injection	Length of Time Since Last Injection		
	No Oral Supplementation Required	Supplement With 7 Days of Oral Aripiprazole	Supplement with 21 Days Oral Aripiprazole
Monthly 441 mg	≤6 weeks	>6 and ≤7 weeks	>7 weeks
Monthly 662 mg	≤8 weeks	>8 and ≤12 weeks	>12 weeks
Monthly 882 mg	≤8 weeks	>8 and ≤12 weeks	>12 weeks
882 mg ever 6 weeks	≤8 weeks	>8 and ≤12 weeks	>12 weeks

Bipolar Disorder, Antiepileptic Drugs & Mood Stabilizers

Antiepileptic drugs (AEDs) have a wide array of uses. They serve in the treatment of several disorders including various treatments of epilepsy, migraines, neuropathy, bipolar disorder and other various illnesses.

This section includes:
- DSM V definition of bipolar disorder and various subtypes
- A general overview of antiepileptic drugs and mood stabilizers
- Classes of medication charts
- Dose form, route and dosage range table
- Pharmacokinetics table
- FDA approved uses table
- Clinical pearls

Bipolar Disorder Subtypes

Bipolar I Disorder
- Made after one manic episode not explained by a diagnosis categorized as a schizophrenia spectrum and/or other psychotic disorder.
- Hypomanic or depressive episode may occur before or after manic episode.

Bipolar II Disorder
- Hypomanic episode and at least one major depressive episode (not explained as a schizophrenia spectrum and/or other psychotic disorder).
- No history of manic episode.
- Depressive/hypomanic episode must cause significant impairment of functioning.

Cyclothymic Disorder
- At least 2 years (1 year in children/adolescents) of numerous periods with hypomanic and depressive symptoms (that do not meet criteria for hypomanic/major depressive episode). The symptoms are not explained by a diagnosis categorized as a schizophrenia spectrum and/or other psychotic disorder.
- Symptoms not attributable to physiological effects of a substance (i.e. drug or abuse or a medication) or another medical condition (i.e. hyperthyroidism).
- At least 50% of time has hypomanic/depressive symptoms and not without symptoms for ≥ 2 months.
- Symptoms must cause significant impairment of functioning.

Bipolar and Related Disorders (*Refer to DSM-V for details*)
- Substance/Medication-Induced Bipolar and Related Disorder.

- Bipolar and Related Disorders Due to Another Medical Condition.
- Other Specified and Related Disorder.

Specifiers for Bipolar and Related Disorders (*Refer to DSM-V for details*)
1. With Anxious Distress
2. With Mixed Features
3. With Rapid Cycling
4. With Melancholic Features
5. With Atypical Features
6. With Psychotic Features
7. With Catatonia
8. With Peripartum Onset
9. With Seasonal Pattern
10. Specifiers for Remission Status or Episode Severity

DIAGNOSTIC CRITERIA (DSM-5)
Bipolar Disorder

Manic Episode

Distinct period (≥ 1 week) of abnormally & persistently elevated, expansive or irritable mood along with abnormally and persistently increased goal-directed activity or energy that is present most of the day, nearly every day or at any duration if hospitalization is necessary.

Minimum of 3 of the following or 4 if mood is only characterized as irritable:

1. Inflated self-esteem or grandiosity
2. Decreased need for sleep (i.e. feels rested after only 3 hours of sleep
3. More talkative than usual or pressure to keep talking
4. Flight of ideas or subjective experience that thoughts are racing
5. Distractibility as reported or observed (attention drawn to unimportant/irrelevant external stimuli)
6. Increase in goal-directed activity (socially, at work/school or sexually) or psychomotor agitation (purposeless non-goal-directed activity)
7. Excessive involvement in activities that have a high potential for painful consequences (i.e. engaging in unrestrained buying sprees, sexual indiscretions or foolish business investments)

Hypomanic Episode

Distinct period of abnormally and persistently elevated, expansive or irritable mood along with abnormally and persistently increased activity or energy, lasting at least 4 consecutive days and present most of the day, nearly every day.

MANIA
DIGFAST
Distractibility
Indiscretion
Grandiosity
Flight of Ideas
Activity Increase
Sleep deficit
Talkativeness

HYPOMANIA
TAD HIGH
Talkative
Attention deficit
Decreased sleep
High self-esteem
Ideas that race
Goal-directed
  activity increased
High-risk activity

Minimum of 3 of the following or 4 if mood is only characterized as irritable:
1. Inflated self-esteem or grandiosity
2. Decreased need for sleep (i.e. feels rested after only 3 hours of sleep
3. More talkative than usual or pressure to keep talking
4. Flight of ideas or subjective experience that thoughts are racing
5. Distractibility as reported or observed (attention drawn to unimportant/irrelevant external stimuli)
6. Increase in goal-directed activity (socially, at work/school or sexually) or psychomotor agitation (purposeless non-goal-directed activity)
7. Excessive involvement in activities that have a high potential for painful consequences (i.e. engaging in unrestrained buying sprees, sexual indiscretions or foolish business investments)

Major Depressive Episode
Five (or more) of the following symptoms have been present during the same 2 week period and represent a change from previous functioning. At least one of the symptoms is either (1) depressed mood or (2) loss of interest or pleasure.
1. Depressed mood most of the day, nearly every day, as indicated by either subjective report (i.e. feels sad, empty or hopeless) or observation made by others (i.e. appears tearful)
2. Markedly diminished interest or pleasure in all, or almost all, activities most of the day, nearly every day (as indicated by either subjective account or observation)
3. Significant weight loss when not dieting or weight gain (i.e. change of ≥ 5% of body weight in a month) or a decrease/increase in appetite nearly every day
4. Insomnia or hypersomnia nearly every day
5. Psychomotor agitation or retardation nearly every day
6. Fatigue or loss of energy nearly every day
7. Feelings of worthlessness or excessive inappropriate guilt (may be delusional) nearly every day
8. Diminished ability to think or concentrate or indecisiveness nearly every day
9. Recurrent thoughts of death (not just fear of dying.) Recurrent suicidal ideation without a specific plan or a suicide attempt or a specific plan for committing suicide[1]

Table 1 describes dosage form, route of administration, and usual daily dose of various medications used for bipolar disorder, epilepsy, and mood stabilization:

Generic Name	Brand Name	Dosage Form*	Route	Dose Range
Anti-Epileptic Drugs (AEDs)				
Carbamazepine	Carbatrol® Carnexiv™ Epitol® Equetro™ Tegretol/XR®	Ch, ERC, ERT, L, SI, T	PO	200-1600 mg
Lamotrigine	Lamictal/CD/ ODT/XR®	Ch, ERT, ODT, T	PO	12.5-400 mg
Divalproex & Valproic Acid	Depacon® Depakene® Depakote/ER®	C, DRC, DRT, ERT, L, SI	PO/IV	125-3000mg *10-60 mg/kg*
NOT FDA APPROVED BUT COMMONLY USED AS ADJUNCTIVE or ADD-ONs				
Gabapentin	Gralise® Horizant® Neurontin®	C, ERT, L, T	PO	100-3600 mg
Oxcarbazepine	Oxtellar XR® Trileptal®	ERT, L, T	PO	300-2400 mg
Topiramate	Qudexy XR® Topamax/ Sprinkle® Topiragen® Trokendi®	C, ERC, T	PO	25-400 mg
Miscellaneous Mood Stabilizers				
Lithium	Eskalith/CR® Lithobid®	C, ERT, T, L	PO	300-2400 mg
Olanzapine + Fluoxetine	Symbyax®	C	PO	3/25-18/75 mg

*C: Capsule, Ch: Chewable, L: Liquid for oral use, DRC: Delayed Release Capsule, ERC: Extended-Release Capsule, ERT: Extended-Release Tablet, ODT: Orally Disintegrating Tablet, SI: Solution/suspension for injection, T: Tablet

Table 2 describes various pharmacokinetic profiles of various medications used for bipolar disorder, epilepsy, and mood stabilization including mechanism of action (MOA), half-life ($t_{1/2}$), and metabolizing/inhibited enzymes:

Drug	MOA #	$T_{1/2}$ (Hours)*	Metabolism^	Enzyme Inhibited^
Aripiprazole	SGA	75; *94*	CYP 3A4 & 2D6	N/A
Asenapine[H]	SGA	24	UGT & CYP 1A2	Weak CYP2D6
Carbamazepine[H]	AED	25-65; Autoinducer after many doses: 12-17	CYP 3A4	Potent Inducer CYP3A4
Cariprazine[H, R]	SGA	2-4 days; 1-3 weeks	CYP 3A4 & 2D6	N/A
Chlorpromazine[H]	FGA	~23-37	CYP 2D6	Moderate Inhibition CYP 2D6
Divalproex[H, R]	AED	9-16	UGT, CYP2A6, 2B6, 2C9, 2C19, 3A4, P-gp	Inhibits UGT & Weak CYP3A4 & 2C19
Gabapentin[R]	AED	5-7	N/A	N/A
Lamotrigine	AED	~24	UGT	N/A
Lithium[R]	Misc	24	N/A	N/A
Loxapine	FGA	4-PO; 12-IM; 7.61 Inhaled	CYP 1A2, 2D6, 3A4 & P-gp	N/A
Lurasidone[H, R]	SGA	18	CYP 3A4	N/A
Olanzapine[H]	SGA	21-54 (Avg 30)	CYP 1A2 & 2D6	N/A
Olanzapine + Fluoxetine[H]	SGA+ SSRI	See individual drugs	See individual drugs	See individual drugs
Oxcarbazepine[H,R]	AED	2; *9*	CYP 3A4/5	Inhibits CYP2C19
Quetiapine[H]	SGA	6 (IR); 7 (ER)	CYP 3A4	N/A
Risperidone[H, R]	SGA	3-24 (PO) 3-6 days (IM)	CYP 2D6	Weak CYP 2D6 inhibitor
Topiramate[H, R]	AED	21	Hydroxylation, Hydrolysis, UGT	N/A
Ziprasidone[H]	SGA	7 (PO) 2-5 (IM)	Glutathione CYP 3A4	N/A

[H]Caution advised in hepatic impairment   [R]Caution advised in renal impairment
[#]SGA: Second Generation Antipsychotic, AED: Antiepileptic drug, SSRI: Selective serotonin reuptake inhibitor. *After Oral Administration. *Italicized is half-life of active metabolite.* ^CYP: Cytochrome, UGT-G: UDP-glucuronosyltransferase-Glucuronidation, P-gp: P-glycoprotein

Table 3 describes FDA approved indications for various drugs:

MEDICATION	BIPOLAR MANIA	BIPOLAR MAINTENANCE	BIPOLAR DEPRESSION	BIPOLAR MIXED EPISODES
Aripiprazole	X [Ψ]	X [Ψ]		X
Asenapine	X [Ψ]			X
Carbamazepine	X			X
Cariprazine	X			X
Chlorpromazine	X			
Lamotrigine		X		
Lithium	X	X		
Loxapine[Ж]	Acute Agitation Bipolar I disorder			
Lurasidone			X [Ψ]	
Olanzapine	X [Ψ]	X		X [Ψ]
Olanzapine + Fluoxetine			X	
Quetiapine/XR	X [Ψ]	X [€]	X	(XR tablet [Ψ])
Risperidone	X [Ψ]	X [Ψ] (IM-Consta [Ψ])		X [Ψ]
Valproate (Divalproex ER)	X			
Ziprasidone	X	X [€]		X
Ψ-Approved for adjunctive and monotherapy €-Approved as adjunctive therapy only				
Ж-Acute agitation Bipolar I disorder				

Clinical Pearls

DRESS (Drug Reaction with Eosinophilia and Systemic Symptoms) has been reported with the following:
- Carbamazepine, Divalproex, Gabapentin, Lamotrigine, Olanzapine, Quetiapine, Ziprasidone[6,7]

FDA Black Box Warning (BBW) regarding all SGAs in treatment of dementia-related psychosis in elderly:
- In April 2005 the FDA mandated that all manufacturers of atypical antipsychotics include a boxed warning to the labeling indicating that increased death rates (1.6—1.7 times that of placebo) have been noted in this patient population receiving atypical antipsychotics. Death typically occurred due to heart failure, sudden death, or infections (primarily pneumonia).[6]
- Refer to Antipsychotic section regarding specific warnings per individual antipsychotic

Monitor for Suicidal Behavior and Ideation with Antiepileptic Drugs.[7]

Dosing below is for Bipolar disorder- dosing may vary for other conditions

Antiepileptic Drugs (AEDs)

<u>MOA</u>: Differs per individual AED—see package insert for details

<u>Adverse Effects:</u> Ranges per individual AED—see listed below med

<u>Contraindications</u>: Ranges per individual AED—see listed below medication

<u>Carbamazepine (Carbatrol®; Carnexiv™; Epitol®; Equetro®; Tegretol/XR®)</u>[19-21]

Available: 100 mg Chewable tablet; 200 mg IR tablets; 100, 200, 400 mg ER tablets; 100 mg, 200 mg, 300 mg ER capsules; 100 mg/5mL Suspension

<u>Dose:</u> 400 mg/day divided BID for XR & QID for IR. Adjust by 200 mg/day; Max dose of 1600 mg/day

<u>Renal:</u> *Caution* in severe renal impairment; *GFR < 10 mL/min:* give 75% of dose. Dialysis-give 75% of dose post-dialysis

<u>Hepatic:</u> Hepatic impairment-use *caution*; metabolized primarily by liver

- Similar structure to TCAs—avoid with MAOI or TCA/CBZ hypersensitivity
- Avoid in bone marrow suppression and pregnancy
- Asian patients should undergo blood test for HLA-B 1502
- Auto-induction occurs 3-5 weeks after initiation of a fixed dose
- Monitor CBC, LFTs, serum carbamazepine level of 4-12 mcg/ml (baseline & 1-2 weeks after each dose change then every 3-6 months thereafter)
- Caution for hyponatremia, leukopenia and elevated LFTs
- Carnexiv™-short-term (≤ 7d) IV use at 70% of total oral dose in 4 ÷ doses
- **POTENT CYP3A4 INDUCER**

<u>Divalproex (Depacon®; Depakene®; Depakote/ER®)</u>[23-26]

Available: 125 mg sprinkle capsules; 125, 250, 500 mg DR tablets; 250,500 mg ER tablets; 250 mg/5ml solution; 100mg/mL IV injection for solution

<u>Dose:</u> 750 mg/day in divided doses titrated rapidly to lowest effective dose

ER: 25-60 mg/kg/day; Max dose of 60 mg/kg/day

<u>Renal:</u> *Severe renal impairment*-uremia can increase free fraction of drug possibly resulting in toxicity. Monitor serum concentrations closely.

<u>Hepatic:</u> Use with *caution* in hepatic impairment; metabolized primarily by liver; contraindicated in severe impairment

- Avoid in hepatic disease, mitochondrial disease or pregnancy
- Monitor CBC, LFTs and serum VPA level (baseline & 1-2 weeks after dose change then every 3-6 months thereafter)
- Caution for thrombocytopenia and elevated LFTs
- VPA trough level 50-100 mcg/mL and up to 125 mcg/mL in acute mania
- Discontinue if pancreatitis is suspected and/or diagnosed
- Quick dosing tool: Weight (lbs) X 10 (i.e. 125 lbs x 10 ~ dose of 1250mg/day)
- ER dose produce concentration fluctuations ~10-20% lower (adjust accordingly)

Gabapentin (Gralise®; Horizant ®; Neurontin®)[27-32]

Available: 100, 300, 400 mg capsules; 100, 300, 400, 600, 800mg tablets; 300, 600 mg ER tablets; 250 mg/5mL oral solution

Dose: Initiate at 300 mg/day titrated up to 2400 mg/day (BID-QID)

Renal: *Caution* adjust accordingly for IR formulations (ER varies slightly). *CrCl 30-59 mL/min:* 200-700mg BID. *CrCl 15-29 mL/min:* 200-700 mg Daily. *CrCl 15mL/min:* 100-300 mg Daily, *CrCl <15mL/min:* reduce in proportion (i.e. for CrCl 7.5 mL/min, use ½ dose of 15 mL/min). *Hemodialysis:* Maintenance dose based upon CrCl with a supplemental post-dialysis dose ranging from 125-350 mg ~4 hours after dialysis

Hepatic: No dose adjustment

- Monitor kidney function
- As dose is increased bioavailability decreased (Gabapentin Bioavailability mg/day-900, 1200, 2400, 3600mg/d ~60%, 47%, 34%, and 33%)
- Not indicated as monotherapy-often added as adjunctive/add-on therapy

Lamotrigine (Lamictal/CD/ODT/XR®)[45-47]

Available: 25, 100, 150, 200 mg IR tablets; 25, 50, 100, 200, 250, 300 mg ER tablets; 25, 50, 100, 200 mg ODT; 5, 25 mg Chewable tablets

Dose: 200 mg/day (See dosing titration below)

Renal: Caution in mild-mod renal impairment. *CrCl 10-50 mL/min:* suggest reduce dose 25%. *CrCl < 10 mL/min:* suggest 100 mg every other day. *Hemodialysis:* 100 mg after dialysis and PD: 100mg every other day.

Hepatic: *Mod-Severe impairment:* reduce dose 25%. *Severe impairment with ascites:* reduce dose 50%.

Medication Titration*:

Week	Monotherapy	With VPA	With EI-AED
1-2	25 mg daily	12.5 mg daily or 25mg QOD	50 mg daily
3-4	50 mg daily	25 mg daily	50 mg BID
5	100 mg daily	50 mg daily	100 mg BID
6 and thereafter	200 mg daily	100 mg daily	150 mg BID WK 6 200 mg BID WK 7
Usual maintenance dose	200-400 mg/day (in 2 ÷ doses)	100-200 mg/day (1-2 ÷ doses)	300-500 mg/day (in 2 ÷ doses)
*VPA: Valproic Acid, CBZ: Carbamazepine, EI-AED: Enzyme-inducing antiepileptic (Carbamazepine, Phenobarbital, Phenytoin, Primidone, Protease Inhibitors, Rifampin, estrogen-containing oral contraceptives), QOD: Every Other Day, WK: week; ÷:divided			

- Slow titration recommended to minimize potential of rash
- If stopped for more than 5 half-lives re-titration is recommended
- Monitor for adverse effects during pill-free week of estrogen-containing oral contraceptives. May need to reduce Lamotrigine dose or consider continuous oral contraceptive.

Oxcarbazepine (Oxtellar XR®; Trileptal®)[35-38]

Available: 150, 300, 600 mg IR tablets; 150, 300, 600 mg ER tablets; 300 mg/5 mL Suspension

Dose: 300 mg BID increased by 300 mg/day every 2 days, max of 2400 mg/day

Renal: *CrCl < 30 mL/min:* start 300 mg/day for 1 week and increase by 300-450 mg/day weekly.

Hepatic: Mild-Mod impairment-no adjustment

Severe impairment-do not administer in severe impairment

- Monitor for hyponatremia (typically within first 3 months; may occur 1 year after treatment initiation)

Topiramate (Qudexy XR®; Topamax/Sprinkle®; Topiragen®; Trokendi®)[62-65]

Available: 25, 50, 100, 200 mg IR tablets; 15, 25 mg capsule; 25, 50, 100, 150, 200 mg ER tablets

Dose: 25-50 mg/day and increase by increments of 25-50 mg/day

Max dose of 400 mg/day

Renal: *CrCl 10-70 mL/min:* decrease dose 50%. *CrCl < 10 mL/min*: decrease dose 75%

Hemodialysis: Supplemental dose may be required post-dialysis

Hepatic: *Caution* advised

- Caution in patients with history of kidney stones
- Titrate slowly to avoid confusion, cognitive impairment and/or word finding difficulties (aka "dopamax")

Miscellaneous Mood Stabilizer

MOA: Competes at cellular sites with sodium, potassium, calcium and magnesium ions. Lithium readily passes through sodium channels and high concentrations can block potassium channels. Evidence suggest that the drug interferes with synthesis, storage, release and reuptake of monoamine neurotransmitters. Enhances uptake of tryptophan, increases synthesis of serotonin, and may enhance release of serotonin in central nervous system.

Adverse Effects: Drowsiness, leukocytosis, memory impairment, polydipsia, polyuria, teratogenesis, tremor, weight gain, xerosis (most common adverse event). May exacerbate psoriasis and/or acne.

Contraindications: *Precaution in cardiac, renal, seizure and thyroid disease.* Avoid in pregnancy and breast feeding.

Lithium (Eskalith/CR®; Lithobid®)[48-52]

Available: 150, 300, 600 mg capsules; 300, 450 mg ER tablets; 300 mg/5mL Solution

Dose: Start at 600-900 mg/day divided BID-TID may increase by 300 mg/day weekly until 1200 mg/day and may further increase by 150-300 mg/day weekly. Typical dosing is 900-1200 mg/day divided TID-QID. *Usual* max Dose of 2400 mg/day (1800 mg/day for ER)

Renal: Caution in mild-mod renal impairment; Contraindicated in severe impairment. *CrCl 10-50 mL/min:* decrease dose 25-50% *CrCl <10mL/min:* decrease dose 50-75% CAUTIOUS USE.

Hemodialysis: dose after dialysis

Hepatic: No adjustment

- TOXIC IN OVERDOSE—NARROW THERAPUETIC WINDOW
- Avoid in severe cardiovascular disease-baseline EKG recommended; may result in abnormal T waves
- TSH (baseline & every 6 months), SrCr & Li level (baseline & 1 week after dose change then every 3-6 months as clinically indicated)
- Serum levels drawn as trough (12 hours post dose) with steady state (SS) occurring 5-7 days after dose change
  - Acute phase 0.8-1.2 meq/L
  - Maintenance phase 0.4-1.0 meq/L
  - Avoid plasma concentrations above 1.5 meq/L
- Lithium Carbonate 300mg typically results in increase of plasma concentration by ~ 0.2-0.4 meq/L in adults
- ER tablet-slower absorption, lower peak, lower bioavailability
- Levels may be affected by water balance, sodium balance, renal function
- Drug interactions: ACEI/ARBs, diuretics, NSAIDs
- Leukocytosis peaks within 7-10 days. WBC % returns to baseline 7-10 days after discontinuation

First Generation Antipsychotics (FGAs)

Chlorpromazine (Thorazine®)[22]

Available: 10, 25, 50, 100, 200 mg tablets; 25 mg/mL IM or IV

Dose: 10-25 mg TID with increase of 25-50 mg/day

Usual dose of 200-800 mg/day divided BID-QID with max of 1000 mg/day

Renal: No adjustment necessary

Hepatic: *Caution* advised

Loxapine (ADASUVE®; Loxitane®)[39-40]

Available: 5, 10, 25, 50 mg capsules; 10 mg/actuation Dry Powder Inhaler

Dose: 10 mg puff inhaled every 24 hours as needed

Renal: No adjustment necessary

Hepatic: No adjustment necessary

- Contraindicated in patients with current diagnosis or history of asthma, COPD or other pulmonary disease associated with bronchospasm
- Administration of inhaled Loxapine requires specialized care setting with immediate on-site access to supplies and personnel trained to manage acute bronchospasm and ready access to emergency response services
- **REMS DRUG (ADASUVE®)** Restricted Distribution in US: 1-855-755-0492 or www.adasuverems.com[60]

Discontinue if ANC < 1000/mm^3 or consider discontinuation if unexplained decrease in WBC.

Metabolic monitoring parameters per ADA & APA consensus guidelines[8]:

	Baseline	Week 4	Week 8	Quarterly	Annually
Medical History[1]	X			X	X
Weight (BMI)	X	X	X	X	X
Waist circumference	X			X	X
Blood pressure	X			X	X
Fasting glucose	X			X	X
Fasting lipids	X			X	X

[1]*Personal & family history of obesity, diabetes, hypertension and cardiovascular disease*

Aripiprazole (Abilify/Discmelt®; Abilify Maintena®; Aristada®)[9-16]

Available: 2, 5, 10, 15, 20, 30 mg tablets; 10, 15 mg ODT; 1 mg/mL Oral Solution; 300, 400 mg ER suspension for injection; 441mg/1.6ml, 662mg/2.4ml and 882mg/3.2ml ER suspension for injection

Dose: 15 mg QDAILY (monotherapy) or 10-15 mg QDAILY (adjunctive)

Max: 30 mg/day

DECREASE DOSE 50% IN POOR CYP2D6 METABOLIZERS OR IF COMBINED WITH STRONG CYP2D6 OR 3A4 INHIBITORS

Renal: No adjustment necessary

Hepatic: No adjustment necessary

- Long half-life. No need to dose more than QDAILY; Steady state ~2 weeks
- Warnings of new onset impulse-control issues

Asenapine (Saphris®)[17]

Available: 2.5, 5, 10 mg sublingual (SL) tablets

Dose: 10 mg SL BID; Max: 20 mg/day

Renal: No adjustment necessary

Hepatic: *Child-Pugh Class A or B*: no adjustment. *Child-Pugh Class C*: contraindicated (average exposure 7x higher)

- Drinking water 2 or 5 minutes after administration reduced exposure by 19% and 10%, respectively
- Avoid eating/drinking 10 minutes after administration
- SL dosing (~35% bioavailable) decreased to <2% is swallowed
- Oral hypoesthesia may occur (typically resolves within 1 hour)

Available: 1.5, 3, 4.5, 6 mg capsules

Dose: 1.5 mg/day; may be increased to 3 mg/day on day 2 with further dose adjustments by 1.5-3 mg/day. Usual dose 3-6 mg/day. Max dose: 6 mg/day

Renal: *Caution* in mild-mod renal impairment; *contraindicated* in severe renal impairment (*CrCl < 30 mL/min*: do not use)

Hepatic: *Mild-moderate (Child-Pugh 5-9):* no adjustments

Severe hepatic (Child-Pugh 10-15:) Do not use—not evaluated. Contraindicated in patients with abnormal LFTs, hepatic impairment or history of liver disease

- Long T ½ so clinical response following dose change may be delayed
- **STRONG 3A4 INHIBITORS MAX DOSE 3MG/DAY—SEE PI FOR DOSING**

Lurasidone (Latuda®)[60]

Available: 20, 40, 60, 80, 120 mg tablets

Dose: Initially 20 mg/day titrated up as tolerated Max Dose: 120 mg/day

Renal: *CrCl > 50 ml/min:* no adjustment. *CrCl < 50 mL/min:* initially 20 mg/day not to exceed 80 mg/day

Hepatic: **Mild impairment:** no adjustments. **Moderate impairment (Child Pugh 7-9):** initially 20 mg/day not to exceed 80 mg/day. **Severe impairment (Child Pugh 10-15):** initially 20 mg/day not to exceed 40 mg/day

- Administer with food (at least 350 calories)
- **CONTRAINDICATED WITH STRONG 3A4 INHIBITORS/INDUCERS**
- **REDUCE BY 50% WITH MODERATE 3A4 INHIBITORS**
- Higher dose 80-120 mg/day did not provide additional benefit over lower dose of 20-60 mg/day

Olanzapine (Zyprexa/Zydis®; Zyprexa Relprevv™)[53,55,56,58]

Available: 2.5, 5, 7.5, 10, 15, 20 mg tablets; 5, 10, 15, 20 mg ODT; 10 mg/vial (5 mg/ml) IR injection; 210, 300, 405 mg ER powder/suspension injection

Dose: 10-15 mg/day with adjustments of 5 mg/day every 24 hours

Max dose: **Oral:** 20 mg/day; **IM:** 10mg IM initially; may repeat after 2hr then again after 4hrs for Max of 30 mg/day

Renal: No dose adjustment

Hepatic: Clearance may be *impaired* in severe hepatic dysfunction

- Clearance 40% higher in smokers (CYP1A2 induction) than nonsmokers
- Typically weight gain is severe

Olanzapine + Fluoxetine (Symbyax®)[54,57]

Available: 3/25, 6/25, 6/50, 12/25, 12/50 mg capsules

Dose: 6/25 mg/day and adjust dose if indicated/tolerated

Max Dose: 18/75 mg

Renal: No dose adjustment

Hepatic: Initially 3/25 mg increased as tolerated

<u>Quetiapine (Seroquel/XR®)</u>[69-70]

Available: 25, 50, 100, 200, 300, 400 mg tablets; 50, 150, 200, 300, 400 mg Extended Release Tablets

<u>Dose:</u> **IR tablets:** 50 mg BID day 1 and increase in increments of 100 mg/day as tolerated to 400 mg/day by day 4. May further increase to 800 mg/day by day 6. **ER/XR tablets:** 300 mg/day on day 1 followed by 600 mg/day on day 2. Max of 800 mg/day both regular and extended release tablets.

<u>Renal:</u> No dose adjustment needed with *CrCl > 10 ml/min*

<u>Hepatic:</u> Hepatic impairment results in 30% *reduced clearance*

- Usually dose at bedtime due to sedation. Slow titration in patients with risk of hypotension. If off for > 1 week follow initial titration.
- REDUCE DOSE 1/6th OF ORIGINAL DOSE WITH POTENT 3A4 INHBITORS
- MAY NEED TO INCREASE DOSE 5-FOLD WITH POTENT 3A4 INDUCERS
- XR version had statistically significant increases in Cmax & AUC with high-fat meal (800-1000 calories) but no significant effect with light meal of 300 calories. XR should be given WITHOUT FOOD or LIGHT MEAL ONLY

<u>Risperidone (Risperdal/M-Tab®; Risperdal Consta®)</u>[66-67]

Available: 0.25, 0.5, 1, 2, 3, 4 mg tablets; 0.25, 0.5, 1, 2, 3, 4 mg Orally disintegrating tablets (ODT); 1 mg/1 ml oral solution; 12.5, 25, 37.5, 50 mg powder for solution injection

<u>Dose:</u> **PO**: Initially 2-3 mg/day adjust by 1 mg/day every 24 hours. **IM**: 25 mg IM every 2 weeks with upward adjustments every 4 weeks. Max of 6 mg/day and 50 mg IM every 2 weeks in Bipolar Disorder.

<u>Renal:</u> *Several renal impairment CrCl < 30ml/min:* lower initial dose of 0.5 mg BID may adjust by 0.5 mg BID as tolerated

<u>Hepatic:</u> *lower* initial dose of 0.5 mg BID may adjust by 0.5 mg BID

- IM injections require established PO dosing of molecule prior to LAI
- IM injections require PO overlap of 3 weeks
- **CYP2D6 INHIBITORS MAY REDUCE CLEARANCE**

<u>Ziprasidone (Geodon®)</u>[43]

Available: 20, 40, 60, 80 mg capsules; 20 mg powder for solution injection

<u>Dose:</u> Initially 40 mg BID increased to 60-80 mg BID day 2. **IM**: 10-20 mg every 2 hours or 20 mg every 4hrs. Max dose: 160 mg/day or 40 mg/day IM

<u>Renal:</u> No dose adjustments

<u>Hepatic:</u> AUC and half-life may increase in cirrhosis

- **ABSORPTION INCREASED UP TO TWO-FOLD WITH FOOD**
- **Administer with food (at least 500 calories)**
- Avoid in patients with congenital long QT syndrome along with other drugs known to prolong QT interval. Discontinue in any patient with persistent QT interval > 500msec

Attention Deficit Hyperactivity Disorder
Narcolepsy/Somnolence

The psychostimulants (amphetamines and non-amphetamines) are generally used for attention deficit hyperactivity disorder (ADHD) by improving attention span, decreased distractibility, increased ability to follow directions/commands or complete tasks and decreased impulsivity and aggression. They can also be used for other conditions like binge eating disorder (BED), narcolepsy, obesity, traumatic brain injury (TBI), and others.

This section includes:
- DSM-V diagnostic criteria and signs/symptoms of ADHD
- General overview of psychostimulants (amphetamines and non-amphetamines,) and non-stimulants
- FDA approved uses
- Clinical pearls

DIAGNOSTIC CRITERIA (DSM-5)

Attention -Deficit/Hyperactivity Disorder (ADHD)

Characterized by persistent pattern or inattention and/or hyperactivity-impulsivity ≥ 6 months that interferes with functioning or development as characterized by (A) and/or (B):

A. Inattention- 6 or more of the following symptoms (5 or more symptoms if ≥ 17 years old) persists and negatively impact social, academic and/or occupational functioning and is inconsistent with developmental level.
   1. Fails to give close attention to details or makes careless mistakes (schoolwork, work or during other activities.)
   2. Difficulty sustaining attention in tasks or play activity
   3. Does not seem to listen when spoken to directly
   4. Does not follow through on instructions and fails to finish school work, chores or work duties (loses focus, side-tracked, etc.)
   5. Difficulty organizing tasks and activities
   6. Avoids, dislikes or is reluctant to engage in tasks that require sustained mental efforts (school work, homework, etc.)
   7. Loses items necessary for tasks or activities (pencils, books, tools, wallet, keys, paperwork, eyeglasses, mobile telephones, etc.)
   8. Easily distracted by external stimuli
   9. Forgetful in daily activities

B. Hyperactivity and Impulsivity
   1. Fidgets with or taps hands/feet or squirms in seat
   2. Leaves seat in situations when remaining seated is required
   3. Runs about or climbs in situations where it is unacceptable (maybe limited to restlessness in adolescents)

    4.   Difficulty playing or engaging in leisure activities quietly
    5.   Is often "on the go" acting as if "driven by a motor"
    6.   Talks excessively
    7.   Blurts out answers before questions have been completed
    8.   Has difficulty waiting his/her turn

- Several symptoms present before age 12 and are present in two or more settings and there is clear evidence that the sxs interfere with or reduce the quality of social, academic or occupational functioning.
- Symptoms are not solely a manifestation of oppositional behavior, defiance, hostility, or failure to understand instructions or tasks and do not occur exclusively during the course of schizophrenia or another psychotic or mental disorder.
- Three ADHD presentations may be diagnosed based on predominant sx appearance:
  1. Combined presentation: criteria met for (A) and (B) above
  2. Predominately inattentive presentation: criteria only met for (A) and not (B).
  3. Predominately hyperactive/impulsive presentation: criteria only met for (B) and not (A).

> *Update: DSM-IV changes across entire life span, instead of just children. Age of onset has been changed. Subtypes replaced with presentation specifiers. Comorbid diagnosis with autism spectrum disorder is not allowed. Symptom threshold for adults changed from 6 → 5.* [1]

Signs & Symptoms of ADHD

Infant
- Difficulty being soothed—fidgety, irritable, crying, and/or colic
- Feeding issues-poor sucking, crying during feedings, frequent need to feed or difficulty settling into a sucking rhythm
- Short periods or very little sleep
- Constant motion (when mobile/crawling)

School Age
- Unable to stay seated, irritable, explosive, constantly "on the go"
- Not able to play quietly or politely with other children
- Easily distracted; unable to complete tasks or follow directions; appears to not listen
- Impulsive, unable to wait turn, blurts out answers, needs instant gratification
- May appear accident prone due to hyperactivity and impulsivity
- Disorganized-constantly forgetting/losing homework or other important items

Adolescence
- Disorganized, procrastinates, forgetful, inattentive and over reactive
- Reckless driving and risky behavior

Lifestyle and home remedies

- Make a list of tasks and break down tasks into smaller/manageable steps
- Use sticky pads to write notes. Place in/on places that will benefit from a reminder
- Keep appointment book or electronic calendar to track appointments and deadlines
- Take time to set up systems (electronics and/or paper documents) to file and help organize information- use systems regularly to develop routine/habit
- Follow routine and keep items (keys, wallet, electronics, etc) in same place[2]

Table 1 describes dosage form, route of administration, and usual daily dose of various amphetamine stimulants, non-amphetamine stimulants, and non-stimulants:

Generic Name	Brand Name	Dosage Form*	Route	Dose Range
Amphetamine Stimulants				
Amphetamine	Adzenys XR-ODT™	XR-ODT, L	PO	3.1-18.8 mg
	Dyanavel XR™			2.5-20 mg
Amphetamine Sulfate	Evekeo®	T	PO	2.5-60 mg
Amphetamine Salts (Mixed)	Adderall/XR®	ERC, T	PO	2.5-60 mg
Amphetamine Stimulants				
Dextro-amphetamine	Dexedrine/ Spansule® Dextrostat® ProCentra® Zenzedi®	ERC, T, L	PO	5-60 mg IR 10-60 mg XR
Lisdexamfetamine Dimesylate	Vyvanse®	C	PO	10-70 mg
Methamphetamine	Desoxyn®	T	PO	5-25 mg
Non-Amphetamine Stimulants				
Dexmethyl-phenidate	Focalin/XR®	ERC, T	PO	5-20 mg IR 10-40 mg XR
Methylphenidate	Aptensio XR® Concerta® Daytrana® Metadate CD/ER® Methylin/ER® QuilliChew ER™ Quillivant XR® Ritalin/LA/SR®	ERC, ERT, L, T, TP	PO, TP	5-72 mg (SEE BELOW PEARLS FOR DETAILS)

Generic Name	Brand Name	Dosage Form*	Route	Dose Range
Non-Stimulants				
Armodafinil	Nuvigil®	T	PO	150-250 mg
Bupropion	Aplenzin® Budeprion SR/XL® Buproban® Forfivo XL® Wellbutrin/SR/XL® Zyban®	T, ERT	PO	Aplenzin: 174-522 mg Others: IR:200-450mg SR:100-400mg XL:150-450mg
Clonidine	Catapres® Kapvay®	T, ERT	PO	0.05-0.4mg
Guanfacine	Intuniv™ Tenex®	ERT, T	PO	1-4mg
Modafinil	Provigil®	T	PO	200-400mg
Sodium Oxybate	Xyrem®	L	PO	4.5-9 grams

*C: Capsule, L: Liquid for oral use, ERC: Extended-Release Capsule, ERT: Extended-Release Tablet, T: Tablet, TP: Transdermal Patch

Table 2 describes various pharmacokinetic profiles of amphetamine stimulants, non-amphetamine stimulants, and non-stimulants, including mechanism of action (MOA), half-life ($t_{1/2}$) and metabolizing/inhibited enzymes:

Drug	MOA[#]	$T_{1/2}$ (Hours)*	Metabolism[^]	Enzyme Inhibited
Armodafinil [H, R]	Un-known[a]	15	CYP 1A2, CYP 3A4/5, CYP 2C19, P-gp	Induce 1A2 & 3A4/5; Inhibit 2C19
Atomoxetine[H]	NRI	5-8 19-24 (PM)	CYP 2D6	N/A
Amphetamines	AMPH	10-12	CYP 2D6	N/A
Amphetamine Salts (Mixed)	AMPH	6-12 years old: 9-11 13-17 years old: 11-14 Adults: 10-13	CYP 2D6	N/A
Bupropion [H, R]	See "Antidepressant" section for details			
Dextro-amphetamine	AMPH	10-12 (A) 6-8 (C)	CYP 2D6	N/A
Clonidine [H, R]	Alpha-2 Agonist	12-16	Liver	N/A
Dexmethy-lphenidate	STIM	2-4.5	Liver (De-esterification)	N/A
Dextro-amphetamine	AMPH	10-12	Liver	N/A

81

Drug	MOA[#]	T$_{1/2}$ (Hours)*	Metabolism^	Enzyme Inhibited
Guanfacine [H, R]	Alpha-2 Agonist	Age dependent: 10-30 (Shorter T$_{1/2}$ in younger. Longer T$_{1/2}$ in older)	CYP 3A4	N/A
Lisdex-amfetamine	AMPH	10-12	Prodrug conversion (see below)	N/A
Meth-amphetamine	AMPH	4-5	Liver Demethylated	N/A
Methyl-phenidate	STIM	1.3-7.7	Liver (De-esterification)	N/A
Modafinil [H, R]	Un-known[a]	15	CYP 2B6, CYP 3A4, CYP 2C9/19, P-gp	Weak inducer of CYP 3A4
Sodium Oxybate [H]	Un-known	0.5-1	CYP 450	N/A

[H] Caution advised in hepatic impairment   [R] Caution advised in renal impairment

[#] STIM: sympathomimetic/stimulant, AMPH: amphetamine stimulant, NRI: norepinephrine reuptake inhibitor, [a] Binds to dopamine transporter (inhibits reuptake) + Alpha-1 Antagonism, * After Oral Administration, PM: poor metabolizer

^ CYP: Cytochrome, UGT-G: UDP-glucuronosyltransferase-Glucuronidation, P-gp: P-glycoprotein

Table 3 describes FDA approved indications for various drugs:

Drug	FDA Approved Indications*				
	ADHD	Narc-olepsy	Shift Work Sleep D/O	OSA/ Hypopnea Syndrome	Misc
Armodafinil		X	X	X	
Atomoxetine	X				
Amphetamine Sulfate	X	IR tablet			Obesity
Amphetamine Salts (Mixed)	X	IR tablet			
Bupropion	*Off-label*				See AD section
Clonidine	X				HTN; Severe pain
Dexmethylphenidate	X				
Dextroamphetamine	X	X			
Guanfacine	ER tablet				HTN
Lisdexamfetamine	X				BED
Methamphetamine	X	*Off-label*			Obesity
Methylphenidate	X	X			
Modafinil	*Off-label*	X	X	X	
Sodium Oxybate		X			Cata-plexy
*ADHD: Attention Deficit Hyperactivity Disorder, OSA: Obstructive Sleep Apnea, BED: Binge-eating disorder, D/O: disorder, AD: antidepressant, HTN: hypertension					

Clinical Pearls

CNS stimulants
(amphetamines & methylphenidate containing products)
WARNINGS AND PRECAUTIONS

- High potential for abuse and dependency-Black Box Warning (BBW) High Abuse Potential, Dependency.[11-14,16-25, 27-36] MONITOR ACCORDINGLY.

- May cause an increase in blood pressure (average increase of 2-4 mm/Hg) and heart rate (average increase of 3-6 bpm)-though may vary per patient-monitor.[4]

- May cause psychotic or manic symptoms in patients with no prior history, or exacerbation of symptoms in patients with pre-existing psychiatric illness.[7]

- May result in sudden death, stroke and/or myocardial infarction. Avoid in patients with known structural cardiac abnormalities, cardiomyopathy, serious cardiac arrhythmias, coronary artery disease, or other serious cardiac problems.[4,6]

- Have been associated with weight loss & slowing of growth rate in pediatric patients.[58,61] (Monitor height & weight accordingly).

- May result in peripheral vasculopathy and Raynaud's phenomenon. [11-14,16-25, 27-36]

Amphetamine Stimulants[11-21]

MOA: Inhibit reuptake and increase release of Norepinephrine and Dopamine in extraneuronal space (sympathomimetic)

Adverse Effects: agitation, anxiety, bruxism, emotional lability, headache, hypertension, insomnia, loss of appetite, mydriasis, tachycardia, vomiting, nervousness, nausea, weight loss, xerostomia

Contraindications: Avoid use in patients with known structural cardiac abnormalities, cardiomyopathy, serious heart arrhythmia or coronary heart disease.

- Amphetamines are often racemic compounds (l-amphetamine & d-amphetamine). The average elimination half-life ($T_{1/2}$) ranges from 9.77-11 hours for d-amphetamine and 11.5-13.8 hrs for l-amphetamine.
- Amphetamine, as the racemic form, differs from dextroamphetamine:
  - l-isomer is more potent than d-isomer in cardiovascular activity.
  - l-isomer is less potent than d-isomer in causing CNS excitatory activity
  - Racemic form less effective than dextroamphetamine as appetite suppressant

- May be referred to as "anorectics" or "anorexigenics"
- Acidifying and Alkalinizing Agents can alter urinary pH and alter blood levels of amphetamines. Acidifying agents can decrease amphetamine blood levels by increasing clearance whereas alkalinizing agents can increase amphetamine blood levels by reducing urinary elimination. [59]

Amphetamine (Adzenys XR ODT™) [14-15]
Available: 3.1, 6.3, 9.4, 12.5, 15.7, 18.8 mg ER-ODT tablets
Dose: Start at 6.3 mg every morning; Max dose is 18.8 mg for 6-12 years of age, and 12.5 mg for 13-17 years of age
Renal: No change
Hepatic: No change
- *ADZENYS XR-ODT™ contains 3 to 1 ratio of d- to l-amphetamine*
- 50% IR & 50% ER for once daily dosing
- Allow tablet to disintegrate in saliva then swallow
- Tablet should remain in blister pack until patient ready to take it. DO NOT PUSH THROUGH THE FOIL rather tear along perforation, bend the blister where indicated and peel back blister backing accordingly
- DO NOT SUBSTITUTE for other amphetamine on a milligram to milligram basis.
- Patients taking Adderall XR® may be switched to Adzenys XR-ODT™
- Dose equivalency:

Adzenys XR-ODT™	3.1 mg	6.3 mg	9.4 mg	12.5 mg	15.7 mg	18.8 mg
Adderall XR®	5 mg	10 mg	15 mg	20 mg	25 mg	30 mg

Amphetamine (Dyanavel XR™) [16]
Available: 2.5 mg/mL suspension
Dose: Initiate at 2.5 or 5mg QAM; May be increased in increments of 2.5-10mg per day every 4-7 days; Max dose of 20mg/day.
Renal: No change
Hepatic: No change
- *DYANAVEL XR contains d-amphetamine & l-amphetamine- ratio of 3.2 to 1*
- DO NOT SUBSTITUTE for other amphetamine on a mg to mg basis
- Before administering dose—SHAKE BOTTLE

Amphetamine Salts (Adderall/XR®) [11-13]
Available: 5, 7.5, 10, 12.5, 15, 20, 30 mg tablets; 5, 10, 15, 20, 25, 30 mg ER capsules
Dose: 5-60 mg/day (QDaily-TID)
Renal: No change
Hepatic: No change
- *Contains D-amphetamine & L-amphetamine salt-ratio of 3:1*

- ER capsule is 50% IR & 50% DR beads (mimics BID dosing)
- Adderall IR BID (total dose) equivalent to daily dose Adderall XR QAM (i.e. 5mg IR BID → 10mg XR QAM OR 10mg IR BID → 20mg XR QAM)

Amphetamine Sulfate (Evekeo®)[46]
Available: 5, 10 mg tablets
Dose: 5mg QAM-BID; increase by 5mg/day QWK. Give in divided doses at every 4-6 hours. Doses >40mg/day rarely more effective. Max dose in narcolepsy is 60mg/day.
Renal: No change
Hepatic: No change
- *Contains D-amphetamine & L-amphetamine-ratio of 1:1*
- Additional indication for obesity (short-term tx)

Dextroamphetamine (Dexedrine®; ProCentra®; Zenzedi®)[17,18,21]
Available: 2.5, 5, 7.5, 10, 15, 20, 30 mg tablets; 5, 10, 15 mg ER capsules; 5mg/5ml (1 mg/mL)
Dexedrine® 5, 10 mg tablets
Dexedrine Spansule® 5, 10, 15 mg ER capsules
ProCentra® 5mg/5ml (1mg/ml) oral solution
Zenzedi® 2.5, 5, 7.5, 10, 15, 20, 30mg tablets
Dose: 5-60 mg/day (QDAILY-TID); increase by 5-10mg/day QWK
Renal: No change
Hepatic: No change
- Spansule capsule is 50% IR & 50% DR beads

Lisdexamfetamine (Vyvanse®)[20]
Available: 10, 20, 30, 40, 50, 60, 70 mg capsules
Dose: 30-70 mg QAM; increase by 10-20 mg/day weekly
Renal: Caution in mild-mod renal impairment; *glomerular filtration rate (GFR) 15 mL/min to less than 30ml/min* max dose of 50 mg/day; *GFR less than 15mL/min* max dose of 30 mg/day; End stage renal disease (ESRD) max dose of 30 mg/day
Hepatic: No change
- Continuous-release capsule
- Prodrug of Dextroamphetamine—conversion to Dextroamphetamine and L-lysine occurs in blood due to high hydrolytic activity of red blood cells (RBCs).

Methamphetamine (Desoxyn®)[19]
Available: 5 mg tablets
Dose: 20-25 mg/day (QDAILY-BID); increase by 5 mg/day weekly
Renal: No change
Hepatic: No change

Non-Amphetamine Stimulants[22-36]

Psychostimulants work by stimulating CNS activity. Block reuptake and increase release of norepinephrine and dopamine in extraneuronal space (sympathomimetic.) There are cases of painful and prolonged penile erections (priapism) with methylphenidate products (any signs/symptoms require immediate medical attention.)[5]

Dexmethylphenidate (Focalin/XR®) [27]

Available: 2.5, 5, 10 mg tablets;
5, 10, 15, 20, 25, 30, 35, 40 mg ER capsules
Dose: 5-40 mg/day (QDAILY-BID); increase by 5-10 mg/day weekly
Renal: No change
Hepatic: No change

- ER capsule is 50% IR & 50% DR beads (mimics BID dosing)
- Extended release capsules allow for once-daily dosing; biphasic pharmacokinetic profile to provide medication availability all day.

Methylphenidate (Aptensio XR®, Concerta®, Daytrana®, Metadate CD®/ER™, Methylin/ER®, QuilliChew ER™, Quillivant XR®, Ritalin/SR/LA®)[22-26, 28-36]

Available: SEE BELOW
Aptensio XR® 10, 15, 20, 30, 40, 50, 60 mg ER capsules (40%IR/60%CR)
Concerta® 18, 27, 36, 54 mg ER tablets (22%IR/78%CR)
Daytrana® 10, 15, 20, 30 mg/9h patches (9hr patch to hip)
Metadate CD® 10, 20, 30, 40, 50, 60 mg ER capsules (30%IR/70%DR)
Metadate ER™ 20 mg ER tablets
Methylin® 5 mg/5 mL, 10 mg/5 mL Oral Solution (also same as Ritalin)
QuilliChew ER™ 20, 30, 40 mg ER Chewable tablets (30%IR/70%CR)
Quillivant XR® 25 mg/5 mL (5 mg/mL) ER suspension (20%IR/80%DR)
Ritalin® 5, 10, 20 mg tablets; 2.5, 5, 10 mg Chewable tablets
Ritalin LA® 10, 20, 30, 40, 60 mg ER capsules (50%IR/50%DR)
Brand Methylin ER® & Ritalin SR® have been discontinued
Dose: 5-60 mg/day (divided BID-TID with IR versions) 18-72 mg QDAILY ER tablet
Renal: No change
Hepatic: No change

- Multiple formulations as above-biphasic releases mimic once daily dosing
- Apply Daytrana® patch to hip 2 hrs prior to effect; Remove after 9 hours. FDA warning Daytrana®-permanent loss of skin color, chemical leukoderma
- High fat meals may delay peak of stimulant-take 30-45mins before meals
- Quillivant XR® must be shaken vigorously for ≥ 10 secs before giving dose, keep in original container & stable for up to 4 months after reconstituted

- Conversion from Methylphenidate Regimens to Concerta®:

Methylphenidate IR (BID-TID DOSE)	5mg BID-TID	10mg BID-TID	15mg BID-TID	20mg BID-TID
Concerta® (ONCE DAILY DOSE)	18mg QAM	36mg QAM	54mg QAM	72mg QAM

Non-Stimulants

Armodafinil (Nuvigil™)[47]
Available: 50, 150, 200, 250mg tablets
Dose: 150-250 mg QAM
Renal: No change (AUC of inactive metabolite, modafinil acid, increases 9-fold in CrCl ≤ 20 ml/min)
Hepatic: *Severe impairment*; reduce dose

Modafinil (Provigil®)[48]
Available: 100, 200mg tablets
Dose: 200mg QAM with max dose of 400mg QAM
Renal: No change (AUC of inactive metabolite, modafinil acid, increases 9-fold in CrCl ≤ 20ml/min)
Hepatic: *Moderate to severe impairment* decrease dose by 50% (100mg QAM in severe impairment)

Atomoxetine (Strattera®)[44]
Available: 10, 18, 25, 40, 60, 80, 100mg capsules
Dose: 40 QAM x 3 days → 40mg BID (80mg QDAILY) Max of 100 mg/day
Renal: No change
Hepatic: *Moderate impairment (Child-Pugh Class B):* reduce initial & target dose by 50%. *Severe impairment (Child-Pugh Class C):* reduced initial & target dose by 75%
- CYP 2D6 Inhibitors or poor metabolizers start at 40mg QAM for 4 weeks
- May give with food to reduce GI effects
- Do not open capsule as ocular & mucous membrane irritant
- Good option for patients with comorbid anxiety, sleep initiation disorder, substance abuse or tics[57]
- Non-stimulant with no abuse potential, less insomnia and minimal risk of growth effects[61]

Bupropion (Wellbutrin®)[37-43]
Refer to "Antidepressant" section for details

Clonidine (Catapres®) Clonidine ER (Kapvay®)[49-51]

Dose: IR: 0.05 mg/day; increase by 0.05mg evert 3-7 days in 3-4 divided doses

ER: 0.1 mg/day HS; increase by 0.1 mg/day at bedtime every week in 2 divided doses if greater than 0.1 mg/day (if not equal doses—larger dose at bedtime) Max of 0.4 mg/day

Renal: Lower dose may be beneficial- titrate slowly

Hepatic: No change recommended-reduced dose may be considered

- Do not stop abruptly; Taper no more than 0.1 mg/day every 3-7 days
- ER peak concentrations ~50% of IR formulations & ~5hrs later
- Not considered 1st line agent for children due to potential cardiac effects
- Monitor BP at initiation, periodically during treatment & when tapering off
- ER tablets are not interchangeable with IR tablets

Guanfacine (Tenex®) Guanfacine ER (Intuniv™)[52-54]

Dose: ER: 1 mg QD increase by 1 mg/day weekly

Renal: *CrCl < 30ml/min:* may need to adjust dose (50% of drug excreted renally)

Hepatic: *Consider* dose decrease/adjustment (50% of drug is metabolized)

- Do not stop abruptly; Taper dose by 1mg/day every 3-7 days[55]
- Monitor BP & HR at baseline, dose changes and periodically
- Avoid with high fat meals (increases absorption)
- **Decrease Guanfacine ER by ½ with moderately strong CYP 3A4 inhibitor**
- **May increase dose by up to double with mod-strong CYP 3A4 inducer**

Sodium Oxybate (Xyrem®)[45]

Dose: start 2.25 g BID; increase 1.5 g/day weekly; Give 1st dose in bed at HS; 2nd dose 2.5-4 hours later. Dose range: 6-9 g/day in divided doses. Max dose 9 g/day

Renal: No change

Hepatic: *decrease* by 50% to start and titrate to desired effect

- Restricted Distribution in US via REMS and prescribers and patient must enroll and use centralized pharmacy (Xyrem Success Program 1-866-997-3688 or www.xyrem.com)
- Give at least 2 hours after meal
- Contraindicated with barbiturates, alcohol, benzodiazepines, and Z-drugs; use caution with other CNS depressant medications

Tricyclic Antidepressants are considered by many to be second-line agents in the treatment of ADHD and typically used in those who have not responded to stimulants and atomoxetine. The use of TCAs, as in the case of Bupropion, is off label.[56]

Substance Abuse

Opioid Use Disorder (OUD)

Problematic pattern of opioid use leading to clinically significant impairment of distress, manifested by at least two of the following within a 12-month period:

1. Opioids taken in larger amounts or over longer period than intended
2. Persistent desire or unsuccessful efforts to cut down or control opioid use
3. Great deal of time spent seeking to obtain, use or recover from opioid effect
4. Craving, strong desire or urge to use opioids
5. Recurrent opioid use resulting in failure to fulfill major obligations at work, school or home
6. Continued opioid use despite having persistent/recurrent social/interpersonal problems caused by or exacerbated by the effects of opioids
7. Important social, occupational or recreational activities given up or reduced because of opioid use
8. Recurrent opioid use in situations in which it is physically hazardous
9. Continued opioid use despite knowledge of having a persistent or recurrent physical or psychological problem that is likely to have been caused/exacerbated by the substance
10. Tolerance-defined as the following:
    (a) Markedly diminished effect with continued use of same amount of opioid.
    (b) Need for markedly increased amounts of opioids to achieve intoxication/desired effect.
11. Withdrawal as manifested by either:
    a) Opioid withdrawal-defined as 3 (or more) of the following after cessation or reduction in use:
       (1) Dysphoric Mood (2) Nausea or vomiting (3) Muscle Aches (4) Diarrhea (5) Lacrimation or rhinorrhea (6) Yawning (7) Fever (8) Insomnia (9) Pupillary dilation, piloerection or sweating
    b) Opioids (or closely related substance) taken to relieve/avoid withdrawal symptoms

Alcohol Use Disorder (AUD)

A problematic pattern of alcohol use leading to clinically significant impairment or distress manifested by at least 2 of the following within a 12-month period:

1. Alcohol is often taken in larger amounts or over longer period than intended
2. Persistent desire or unsuccessful efforts to cut down or control alcohol use

3. Great deal of time seeking to obtain, use or recover from alcohol effects
4. Craving, strong desire or urge to use alcohol
5. Recurrent alcohol use resulting in failure to fulfill major role obligations at work, school or home
6. Continued alcohol use despite having persistent/recurrent social/interpersonal problems caused or exacerbated by effects of alcohol
7. Important social, occupational or recreational activities given up or reduced because of alcohol use
8. Recurrent alcohol use in situations in which it is physically hazardous
9. Alcohol use continued despite knowledge of having persistent or recurrent physical or psychological problem likely to have been caused/exacerbated by alcohol
10. Tolerance-defined as the following: (a) Markedly diminished effect with continued use of same amount of alcohol. (b) Need for markedly increased amounts of alcohol to achieve intoxication/desired effect.
11. Withdrawal as manifested by either:
    a) Alcohol withdrawal-defined as 2 (or more) of the following after cessation or reduction in use:
    (1) Autonomic hyperactivity (sweating or pulse greater than 100 beats per minute) (2) Anxiety (3) Increased hand tremor (4) Insomnia (5) Nausea or vomiting (6) Transient hallucinations/illusion (auditory, tactile or visual) (7) Psychomotor agitation (8) Generalized tonic-clonic seizures
    b) Alcohol (or closely related substance) taken to relieve/avoid withdrawal symptoms [1]

Urine Drug Screening (UDS)

All UDS results serve as preliminary findings and confirmatory tests (gas chromatography/mass spectrometry (GC/MS)) should be considered if there is doubt or question. As-needed medications will result in variability in UDS results.

Drug	Detection Time in Urine
Amphetamine	Up to 3 days
Benzodiazepines (depends on agent & quantity used)	Days to weeks
Cocaine (Benzoylecgonine metabolite)	2-4 days
Opiates (Codeine, Morphine)	2-3 days
Methadone --EDDP (methadone metabolite)	Up to 3 days --Up to 6 days
THC (depends on frequency of use & grade of marijuana) --Single Use ++Chronic Use	 --1-3 days ++Up to 30 days

A basic UDS will screen for the following:

- **AMPHETAMINES:** HIGHLY false + due to OTC products (diet pills & decongestants), bupropion, selegiline, etc. *Methylphenidate NOT included.*
- **BARBITUARATES:** RELIABLE- Fioricet & Primidone will result in + assay.
- **BENZODIAZEPINES:** Some devices less sensitive for Lorazepam & Clonazepam.
- **CANNABINOIDS:** RARE false positive.
- **COCAINE:** VERY accurate.
- **OPIATES:** does not detect synthetic opioids—see below:
  - *NATURAL:* Codeine, Heroin and Morphine will result in positive assay
  - *SEMI-SYNTHETIC:* Buprenorphine, Hydrocodone, Hydromorphone, Oxycodone and Oxymorphone (Hydrocodone & Hydromorphone may or may not depending upon how much & when dose was taken) others require separate & specific tests.
  - *SYNTHETIC:* Fentanyl, meperidine, methadone, propoxyphene, tapentadol and tramadol will not result in positive UDS, and require separate tests.

False Positive- a falsely positive immunoassay when actual drug wasn't present.
False Negative-a falsely negative immunoassay when actual drug was present but below threshold of detection.

Laboratory devices vary-contact lab for copy of immunoassay sensitivities, thresholds and various medications that may result in cross-reactivity.

Urine Creatinine less than 20 mg/dl and Specific Gravity less than 1.003 should be interpreted with caution as sample may have been adulterated or diluted.

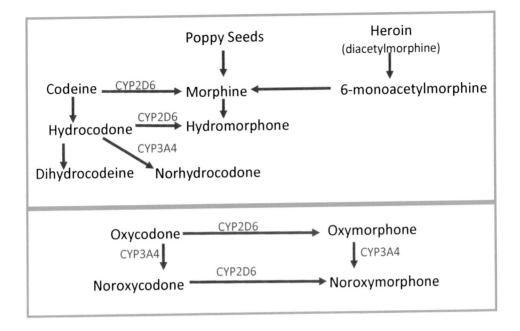

Table 1 describes dosage form, route of administration, and usual daily dose of various medications used in substance abuse:

Generic Name	Brand Name	Dosage Form*	Route	Dose Range
Acamprosate	Campral®	DRT	PO	333-666 mg TID
Buprenorphine	Belbuca™ Buprenex® Butrans® Probuphine® Subutex ®	SDI, SLT, TD, IV/IM, BF	PO, SD	74.2 mg (Implant) 4-24 mg (PO) *Dosing for pain not discussed*

Buprenorphine /Naloxone	Bunavail™
	Suboxone®
	Zubsolv®
		SLT,
		SLF, BF,
		ODT
			PO	Film, buccal:
				  2.1/0.3 mg; 4.2/0.7 mg
				  6.3/1 mg
				Film, sublingual:
				  2/0.5 mg; 4/1 mg
				  8/2 mg; 12/3 mg
				Tablet, sublingual:
				  2/0.5 mg; 8/2 mg
				  0.7/0.18 mg; 1.4/0.36mg
				  2.9/0.71 mg; 5.7/1.4 mg
				  8.6/2.1 mg; 11.4/2.9 mg
				  1.4/0.36-11.4/2.9

Generic Name	Brand Name	Dosage Form*	Route	Dose Range
Disulfiram	Antabuse®	T	PO	250-500mg
Methadone	Dolophine® Methadose®	T, OC, DT	PO	20-120mg
Naltrexone	ReVia® Vivitrol®	T, SI	PO, IM	25-150mg IM: 380mg

*T: Tablet, SI: solution/suspension for injection, BF: buccal film, SLF: sublingual film, SLT: Sublingual tablet, DRT: delayed release tablet, OC: oral concentrate, DT: dispersible tablets, SDI: subdermal implant, TD: Transdermal; IV: Intravenous, IM: Intramuscular, ODT: orally disintegrating tablet

Table 2 describes pharmacokinetic profiles of medications used for substance use disorder, including mechanism of action (MOA), half-life ($t_{1/2}$) and metabolizing/inhibited enzymes:

Drug	MOA	$T_{1/2}$ (Hours)*	Metabolism^	Enzyme Inhibited
Acamprosate[R]	Not fully understood may restore balance of glutamate & GABA	20-33	Does not undergo metabolism	N/A
Bupre-norphine[H]	Partial mu-receptor (μ) agonist Kappa antagonist	PO: 24-42	CYP 3A4, glucuro-nidation	CYP 2D6 & 3A4 Inhibitor
Bupre-norphine/ Naloxone[H]	Partial μ agonist, Kappa antagonist/ μ antagonist	24-42 (BUP) 2-12 (NAL)	CYP 3A4, glucuro-nidation	CYP 2D6 & 3A4 Inhibitor
Disulfiram[H,R]	Aldehyde dehydrogenase inhibitor	12, *15.5*	CYP 1A2, 2A6, 2B6, 2D6, 2E1, 3A4 (all minor)	Inhibits CYP 2E1 & 1A2
Methadone[H,R]	μ agonist, NMDA antagonist	Variable: 8-150	CYP 3A4, 2B6, 2C19 & 2C9	Ch use may Induce 3A4
Naltrexone[H,R]	Pure opioid antagonist	PO: 4-5; *13-14* IM: 5-10 Days	Extensive first pass metabolism	N/A

[H] Caution advised in hepatic impairment   [R] Caution advised in renal impairment
*After Oral Administration Italicized represents $T_{1/2}$ of metabolites, PO: by mouth, IM: Intramuscular, ^CYP: Cytochrome, UGT-G: UDP-glucuronosyltransferase-Glucuronidation

Table 3 describes various FDA approved indications for medications used in substance abuse:

Drug	Alcohol Dependence	Opioid Dependence	Miscellaneous
Acamprosate	X		
Buprenorphine		X	Opiate Agonist Withdrawal & Pain
Buprenorphine/ Naloxone		X	
Disulfiram	X		
Methadone		X	Opiate Agonist withdrawal & Pain
Naltrexone	X	X	

Clinical Pearls

These medications should be used as part of a comprehensive management program that includes psychosocial support.

Buprenorphine products requires Drug Addiction Treatment Act of 2000 (DATA 2000) waiver to provide medication-assisted treatment (MAT) to 30 patients the first year expandable to 100 patients thereafter. Physicians may increase from maximum of 100 opioid-dependent patients to 275 patients if maintained for at least one year without interruption. Restricted distribution in US visit https://www.samhsa.gov/medication-assisted-treatment/physician-program-data/treatment-physician-locator or call 1-866-287-2728. Mid-level practitioners were recently added as per next statement:

Nurse practitioners (NPs) and physician assistants (PAs) can now take the 24-hour training course to prescribe Buprenorphine to treat opioid use disorder. They will be able to apply to be able to prescribe buprenorphine for up to 30 patients in early 2017. The Department of Health and Human Services (HHS) is announcing its intent to initiate rulemaking to allow NPs & PAs who have prescribed at the 30-patient limit for up to 1 year to apply for a waiver to prescribe buprenorphine for up to 100 patients.

Visit http://www.samhsa.gov/medication-assisted-treatment for regulations, guidance and a wealth of resources. Refer to http://www.asam.org for national practice guidelines and pocket resources.

Methadone for opioid addiction, detoxification and maintenance programs must be through opioid treatment programs (OTP) certified by the Substance Abuse and Mental Health Services Administration and approved by designated state authority (exception include treatment during inpatient admission or conditions other than opioid addiction and during an emergency period no longer than 3 days during which addiction care by a licensed facility is being sought).

Naloxone should be considered and offered to any/all individuals in MAT program or deemed at risk of opioid overdose. [27,32]

Benzodiazepines are not recommended in combination with opioids. [28]

Acamprosate (Campral®) [7]
Available: **333mg DR EC tablets**
Dose: 666mg TID
Renal: *CrCl 30-50ml/min:* 333mg TID. *CrCl < 30ml/min:* Contraindicated
Hepatic: No adjustment
- Initiate after withdrawal when abstinence achieved
- Used for ETOH dependence & maintenance treatment
- Diarrhea most common side effect; monitor for depression and suicidality

Buprenorphine (Belbuca™; Buprenex®; Butrans®; Probuphine®; Subutex®) [14, 20-27]
Available: **SEE BELOW:**
Belbuca™: **75, 150, 300, 450, 600, 750, 900 mcg buccal strip/film**
Buprenex®: **0.3 mg/ml Solution for injection (IM/IV)**
Butrans®: **5, 7.5, 10, 15, 20 mcg/hr patch**
Probuphine®: **74.2 mg subdermal implant**
Subutex®: **2, 8 mg SL tablet**
Dose: *Opioid dependence, induction treatment* 2-8 mg SL Day 1, then 8-16mg SL daily for 1-2 days then start maintenance treatment
Max dose of 24 mg/day; however, common to see up to 32 mg/day
Renal: No adjustment
Hepatic: *Moderate impairment*: caution advised
Severe impairment: consider dose decrease of 50%
- Begin 8-12 hours after last opioid use or when withdrawal symptoms present
- Swallowing tablets reduces bioavailability
- Subdermal implant is for patients on low-to-moderate doses (≤8 mg/day) with each dose consisting of 4 implants inserted in the inner side of upper arm with intent to be in place for 6 months
- **PROBUPHINE REMS Program** requires special training/certification on insertion & removal of implant
- Butrans®, BelbucaTM and Buprenex® are all utilized for pain disorders

Available: Buprenorphine/Naloxone: 2/0.5 mg, 8/2 mg SL tablets

Bunavail™: 2.1/0.3 mg, 4.2/0.7 mg, 6.3/1 mg buccal strips

Suboxone®: 2/0.5 mg, 4/1 mg, 8/2 mg, 12/3 mg SL strips

Zubsolv®: 1.4/0.36 mg, 2.9/0.71 mg, 5.7/1.4 mg, 8.6/2.1 mg, 11.4/2.9 mg SL tablets

Dose: *Opioid dependence, induction treatment* 2/0.5 mg to 4/1 mg x 1 dose may increase by 2/0.5 mg to 4/1 mg every 2 hours (up to 8/2 mg on Day 1) then give up to 16/4 mg on Day 2 then start maintenance treatment. Max dose of 24/6mg/day; however, common to see pushed to 32/8 mg/day

Renal: No adjustment

Hepatic: *Moderate impairment*: caution advised

Severe impairment: consider dose decrease of 50% or avoid use

Hepatic impairment reduces naloxone clearance more than buprenorphine clearance

- Not bioequivalent to other buprenorphine/naloxone products
- Plasma levels increased with buccal dose: see table 3

Table 4 describes the approximate dose equivalencies between various dosage forms of buprenorphine/naloxone combination:

1.4/0.36 mg SL tab = 2/0.5 mg SL tablet or strip	2.1/0.3 mg buccal strip = 4/1 mg SL tablet or strip	4.2/0.7 mg buccal strip = 5.7/1.4 mg SL tablet OR 8/2 mg SL tablet or strip	6.3/1mg buccal strip = 8.6/2.1 SL tablet OR 12/3 mg SL tablet or strip

Available: 250, 500 mg tablet

Dose: 500 mg every AM for 1-2 Weeks; may reduce to 125-250 mg daily; Max of 500 mg/day

Renal: No adjustment

Hepatic: *Caution advised*-extreme caution with hepatic cirrhosis of insufficiency

- SEVERE Disulfiram-Alcohol reaction (flushing, nausea, hypotension, etc.)
- Contraindicated in severe myocardial disease, coronary occlusion, psychosis, EtOH use or Metronidazole use
- Must be abstinent from EtOH or EtOH containing products (cough syrup, mouthwash, cologne) for > 12 hours
- Avoid EtOH up to 2 weeks after cessation of drug
- Best reserved for highly motivated patients
- Never administer if EtOH intoxication or without patient's full knowledge
- Metallic taste common side effect; monitor for hepatotoxicity

Methadone (Dolophine®; Methadose®) [8-12]

Available: 5, 10 mg tablets and 40 mg dispersible tablets, 5 mg/5 mL, 10 mg/5 mL oral solution and 10 mg/1 mL intensol oral solution or injection (SC, IM, IV)

Dose: 15-30 mg X 1 dose → 5-10 mg every 2-4 hours PRN; Max 40 mg/day on day 1.
Renal: *CrCl < 10 mL/min*: decrease dose by 25-50%.
Hepatic: *Severe impairment*-caution advised

- Restricted to authorized opioid addiction detox/maintenance facilities
- SC, IM, IV use should be used on temporary basis for non-PO inpatient use
- Adjust dose to suppress withdrawal symptoms & stabilize dose x 2-3 days with decreased dose by up to 20% every 24-48 hours; doses greater than 40 mg/day require documentation in short-term detox
- Adjust dose to prevent withdrawal symptoms for 24 hours & stabilize dose for 10-14 days with decreased dose by up to 10% every 10-14 days; doses greater than 100 mg/day require documentation in maintenance treatment
- Maintenance treatment permitted only in FDA-approved program (Opioid Treatment Programs) certified by SAMSHA & registered by the DEA
- Monitor for QT prolongation and respiratory depression

Naltrexone (ReVia®; Vivitrol®) [3-5]

Available: 50 mg tablet; 380 mg IM solution for injection

Dose: **Opioid dependence**- 25 mg x 1, if no withdrawal may be initiated on 50 mg daily thereafter. Alternative dosing of 100mg every-other-day; 150 mg every 3 days; 380 mg IM every 4 weeks. **EtOH dependence**- 50 mg every day or 380 mg IM every 4 weeks
Renal: *CrCl < 50 ml/min*: caution advised
Hepatic: *Child-Pugh Class C*-caution advised
Increase in AUC of ~ 5- and 10-fold in patients with compensated & decompensated liver cirrhosis, respectively.

- Contraindicated in opiate use or positive urine drug screen; must be opioid free for 7-10 days
- Consider naloxone challenge test if risk of withdrawal suspected and if positive for withdrawal DO NOT initiate naltrexone therapy & repeat in 24 hours
  IV- 0.2 mg then observe for 30 seconds; if no withdrawal symptoms, 0.6 mg observe for 20 minutes
  SQ- 0.8 mg then observe for 20 minutes
- Monitor for signs and symptoms of depression, suicidality and hepatotoxicity
- Suggest carry ID card or bracelet to alert medical personnel in emergency
- 50 mg will block pharmacologic effects of 25 mg of IV heroin for ~24 hours
- Remove from fridge ~45 mins prior to preparation—See package insert for Vivitrol for details pertaining to administration

Naloxone (EVZIO®; Narcan®) [29-31]
Available: 0.4 mg/0.4 mL, 0.4 mg/1mL and 1 mg/mL IV/SC/IM; 4 mg/0.1 ml intranasal spray
Dose: 0.4-2 mg SC/IM/IV every 2-3 minutes PRN; **EVZIO®**-0.4 mg SC/IM every 2-3 minutes PRN; NARCAN®- 4 mg intranasal every 2-3 minutes PRN
Renal: No adjustment
Hepatic: No adjustment

- EVZIO® autoinjector has visual and voice guidance for use
- Do not prime Narcan® nasal sprays

Off Label Pharmacotherapy for Opioid Use Disorder

Clonidine*
Initiate 0.1-0.3 mg PO every 6-8 hours with max dose of 1.2 mg/day to assist in management of opioid withdrawal symptoms. APA guidelines suggest initial dose of 0.1mg TID is usually sufficient to suppress signs of opiate withdrawal. May convert to transdermal patch. Clonidine doses are to be tapered and discontinued 7-10 days after cessation of opiate. [32, 47]
See ADHD section for detailed info pertaining to medication

Off Label Pharmacotherapy for Alcohol Use Disorder

Topiramate*
Initiate 50 mg daily; titrate slowly up to 100 mg BID over several weeks
Gabapentin*
Initiate 300 mg daily; increase by 300 mg/day up to 1800 mg/day in divided doses [33]

See Mood Stabilizer Section for detailed info pertaining to medication

Nicotine Use Disorder

Quit Tools: www.smokefree.gov
Quit Line: 1-877-44U-QUIT (877-448-7848) OR 1-800-QUIT-NOW (800-784-8669)
Nicotine Products(Commit®; Habitrol®; Nicoderm CQ®; Nicotrol® & Nicotrol NS®; Nicorelief®; Nicorette®; ProStep) [34-44]
Available: 2 mg and 4 mg chewing gum
Dose: 4 mg: patients who smoke first cigarette within 30 minutes of waking, 2 mg: patients who smoke first cigarette more than 30 minutes of waking

STEP 1	STEP 2	STEP 3
Weeks 1 to 6	Weeks 7 to 9	Weeks 10-12
1 piece every 1-2 hours	1 piece every 2-4 hours	1 piece every 4-8 hours
DO NOT USE MORE THAN 24 PIECES PER DAY		

Chew gum until tingles, then "park" between cheek and tongue. Once tingle gone, begin chewing until tingle returns. Repeat until tingle gone (~30mins)

Available: 2 mg and 4 mg lozenges

Dose: 4 mg-patients who smoke first cigarette within 30 minutes of waking,
2 mg-patients who smoke first cigarette more than 30 minutes of waking

STEP 1	STEP 2	STEP 3
Weeks 1 to 6	Weeks 7 to 9	Weeks 10-12
1 lozenge every 1-2 hours	1 lozenge every 2-4 hours	1 lozenge every 4-8 hours
DO NOT USE MORE THAN 5 LOZENGES PER 6 HOURS		
DO NOT USE MORE THAN 20 LOZENGES PER 24 HOURS		

Allow lozenge to slowly dissolve in mouth and occasionally move from one side of mouth to the other until completely dissolved (~20-30mins)

Available: 10 mg/mL (0.5 mg actuation nasal spray) & 10 mg/cartridge (4 mg delivered oral inhalation)

Dose: *Nasal:* 0.5 mg/spray in each nostril 1 to 2 times per hour as needed;
Max of 5 doses (10 sprays) per hour & 40 doses (80 sprays) per day.
Prime device by pumping 6-8 sprays into a tissue until a fine mist appears. If not used for more than 24 hours re-prime with 1-2 pumps until mist occurs. Patient to tilt head back slightly, breathe through mouth while dose administered and do not sniff or inhale while administering dose. Do not blow nose for 2-3 minutes following dose. Oral: 24 to 64 mg (6 to 16 cartridges) per day for up to 12 weeks followed by a gradual reduction in dosage over a period of up to 12 weeks. Best results obtained by continuous puffing over ~ 20 minutes. Each cartridge delivers a total of 4mg of nicotine.

Available: 7 mg, 14 mg, and 21 mg transdermal patches

Dose: Per chart

STEP 1	STEP 2	STEP 3
Weeks 1 to 6	Weeks 7 to 9	Weeks 10-12
1 (21mg) patch/day	1 (14mg) patch/day	1 (7mg) patch/day
IF > 10 CIGARETTES/DAY START AT STEP 1		
IF ≤ 10 CIGARETTES/DAY START AT STEP 2		

*Apply patch to hairless area for 16-24 hours. Do not cut or trim patch. Ensure old patch removed before applying new patch-**REMOVE BEFORE MRI**. Habitrol, Nicoderm and ProStep are designed to be worn for 24 hours. Nicotrol is to be applied upon awakening and removed before bed.*

Renal: No adjustment

Hepatic: No adjustment

- Gum/lozenge absorbed buccally and slower than cigarette smoke, inhaled or nasal administration.
- See italicized administration info above for each product

Varenicline (Chantix®) [45]

Available: 0.5 mg and 1 mg tablets

Dose: Titrate dose over the course of 1 week:

0.5 mg daily on days 1-3, then 0.5 mg BID on days 4-7, then 1 mg BID

Patient to pick a quit date and initiate 1 week prior to quit date

Renal: *CrCl of ≤ 30 mL/min:* Initially 0.5 mg daily with max of 0.5 mg BID

Hepatic: No adjustment

- **MOA:** partial agonist at alpha4-beta2 (α4β2) neuronal nicotinic acetylcholine receptors (nAChRs). Produces modest levels of mesolimbic dopamine thus reducing/diminishing nicotine cravings and withdrawal symptoms. Additional benefit of occupying nicotine receptors sites therefore reducing reward of nicotine upon patient relapse of nicotine use.
- T ½ is ~ 24 hours; minimal metabolism and excreted via kidneys
- Common side effects: nausea (~30%), insomnia (~18%), abnormal dreams (~13%), headache (~15%)
- Duration of therapy is 12 weeks; may continue additional 12 weeks if successful
- Black Box Warning for serious mental health adverse reactions removed in December 2016 after FDA reviewed clinical data

Bupropion (Zyban®) [46]

Available: 150 mg sustained release tablets

Dose: 150 mg every morning for 3 days, then 150 mg BID

Initiate 1-2 weeks before "quit date". Separate doses by 8 hours.

See Antidepressant Section for specific details on Bupropion

Weight Loss & Miscellaneous

Medications used for weight loss are known as anorectics or anorexigenics and the use of them has been controversial over the years. Various medications have come and gone as a result of safety concerns (typically cardiovascular though sometimes psychiatric in nature). Fenfluramine (Pondimin®) and Dexfenfluramine (Redux®) were removed from the market in 1997 due to cardiovascular events (heart valve problems) along with pulmonary hypertension. They were commonly used in combination with Phentermine which was known as "Fen-phen". Their mechanism of action was reuptake inhibitor of serotonin 2B receptors.[1,2]

Phenylpropanolamine (PPA) was discontinued in 2000 due to hemorrhagic stroke. It's mechanism of action was alpha and beta adrenergic agonism.[3] Sibutramine (Meridia®) is another medication that was withdrawn from the market in October 2010 due to increased cardiovascular events and strokes. The mechanism of action was SNRI and it was structurally related to amphetamines.[4,5] Since the withdrawal of the above medications there continues to be use of other previously approved medications along with newly approved medications for weight loss.

This section will discuss weight loss medications along with miscellaneous psychiatric medications.

CLINICAL PEARLS

- *Indicated for short-term use of exogenous obesity.*
- Adjunctive treatment regimen to a reduced-calorie diet and increased physical activity for chronic weight management in adults refractory to alternative therapy (i.e. repeated diets, group programs and other drugs) and with a body mass index (BMI) of ≥ 30kg/m^2 (obese), or adults with a BMI of ≥ 27kg/m^2 (overweight) and who have at least 1 weight-related comorbid condition (i.e. hypertension, type 2 diabetes, dyslipidemia).
- Obtain baseline cardiac evaluation in patients with risk factors along with blood pressure and heart rate at baseline, after dose increase and periodically.
- The rate of weight loss is greatest in first weeks of therapy for both drug and placebo subjects and tends to decrease in succeeding weeks.

Table 1 describes various dosage forms, routes of administration, and usual daily dose range for drugs used for weight loss:

Generic Name	Brand Name	Dosage Form*	Route	Dose Range
AMPHETAMINES				
Amphetamine Sulfate	Evekeo®	T	PO	5-30 mg daily
Benzphetamine	Didrex® Regimex™	T	PO	25-150 mg daily
Diethylpropion	Tenuate®/ Dospan®	SRT, T	PO	25 mg TID or 75 mg daily (SR)
METHAMPHETAMINES				
Methamphetamine	Desoxyn®	T	PO	5 mg TID
Phentermine	Adipex-P® Lomaira™	C, T	PO	C: 15-37.5 mg QAM T: 4-8 mg TID
MISCELLANEOUS				
Liraglutide	Saxenda® Victoza®	PFS	SQ	0.6-3 mg daily
Lorcaserin	Belviq®/XR®	ERT, T	PO	10 mg BID or 20 mg daily (XR)
Naltrexone/ Bupropion	Contrave®	ERT	PO	16/180 mg BID
Orlistat	Alli™ Xenical®	C	PO	60-120 mg TID
Phendimetrazine	Bontril PM® Melfiat®	ERC, T	PO	ERC: 150 mg daily T: 17.5-70 mg TID
Phentermine/ Topiramate	Qsymia®	ERC	PO	3.75/23 mg-15/92 mg daily

*C: Capsule, ERC: Extended-Release Capsule, ERT: Extended-Release Tablet, PFS: Pre-Filled Syringe, SR: Sustained Release Tablet, T: Tablet.

Table 2 describes various pharmacokinetic profiles of drugs used for weight loss, including mechanism of action (MOA), half-life ($t_{1/2}$) and metabolizing/inhibited enzymes:

Drug	MOA[#]	T$_{1/2}$ (Hours)*	Metabolism^	Enzyme Inhibited
Amphetamine[R,H]	AMPH	D-amphetamine: 9.77-11 L-amphetamine: 11.5-13.8	CYP2D6	N/A
Benzphetamine	AMPH	7-34	CYP3A4; 2B6	N/A
Diethylpropion[R,H]	SYM	4-6	N-dealkylation & reduction	N/A
Methamphetamine	METH	4-5	CYP2D6; hydroxylation; deamination; N-dealkylation	N/A
Phentermine[R]	METH Analog	19-24	Primarily excreted via kidney	N/A
Liraglutide[R,H]	GLP-1 Agonist	13	Endogenously Metabolized	N/A
Lorcaserin[R,H]	5-HT$_{2C}$ Agonist	IR: 11 ER: 12	Extensive hepatic metabolism	CYP2D6
Naltrexone/ Bupropion[R,H]	Opiate antagonist + DNRI	Naltrexone: 5 Bupropion: 21	CYP2D6 & B6	CYP2D6
Phendimetrazine[R]	SYM	IR: 1.9 ER: 9.8	Primarily excreted via kidney	N/A
Phentermine/ Topiramate[R,H]	METH Analog + AED	Phentermine: 20 Topiramate: 65	CYP 3A4 Hydrolysis, Hydroxylation, Glucuronidation	N/A
Orlistat	Lipase Inhibitor	1-2	Excretion Unchanged	N/A

[R]: Adjust for renal impairment, [H]: Adjust for hepatic impairment.
[#]5-HT$_{2C}$ Agonist: Serotonin 2C agonist, AED: Antiepileptic drug, AMPH: Amphetamine, DNRI: Dopamine Norepinephrine Reuptake Inhibitor, GLP-1: Glucagon-1 Peptide Agonist, METH: Methamphetamine, SYM: Sympathomimetic. *Half-life after oral administration. ^CYP: Cytochrome P450 Enzyme.

AMPHETAMINES

Amphetamine Sulfate (Evekeo®) [6]
Available: 5 and 10 mg tablets
Dose: 5-10 mg ~30-60 minutes before meals. Max of 30 mg/day.
Renal: Use with *caution*; potential for reduced elimination in renal dysfunction.
Hepatic: Use with *caution*; potential for reduced elimination in hepatic dysfunction.

Benzphetamine (Didrex®; Regimex™) [7,8]
Available: 25 mg and 50 mg tablets
Dose: 25-50 mg daily titrated to 25-50 mg TID.
Renal: No adjustment
Hepatic: No adjustment
- Evaluate response to therapy after 4 weeks for satisfactory weight loss (i.e. weight loss of ≥ 4lbs or as determined by physician and patient).

Diethylpropion (Tenuate®/Dospan®) [9]
Available: 25 mg tablet and 75 mg sustained release tablet
Dose: 25 mg TID or 75 mg sustained release every morning.
Renal: No dosing recommended but *caution* advised as excreted renally.
Hepatic: No dosing recommended but *caution* advised.
- Discontinue if no response within 4 weeks or if tolerance occurs.
- Short-term (up to 12 weeks). Longer periods (up to 25 weeks) may be safely and successfully utilized without development of tolerance.
- Structurally similar to Bupropion; sympathomimetic with pharmacologic properties similar to amphetamines.

Phendimetrazine (Bontril PDM®; Melfiat®) [10,11]
Available: 35 mg tablet and 105 mg extended release capsules
Dose: 17.5-35 mg BID-TID about 1 hour before each meal OR 105 mg extended release capsule every morning. Max of 70 mg TID.
Renal: Use with *caution*; phendimetrazine excreted renally.
Hepatic: No adjustment
- Sympathomimetic with pharmacologic properties similar to amphetamines.

METHAMPHETAMINE

Methamphetamine (Desoxyn®) [12,13]
Available: 5 mg tablet
Dose: 5mg about 30 minutes before each meal (5 mg TID).
Renal: No adjustment.
Hepatic: No adjustment.

METHAMPHETAMINE ANALOG

Phentermine (Adipex-P®; Lomaira™) [14-18]

Available: 15 mg, 18.75 mg, 30 mg, 37.5 mg capsules; 8 mg & 37.5 mg tablets

Dose: Lomaira™: 4 mg TID in those with cardiac, hepatic or renal dysfunction; otherwise, 8 mg TID or Adipex-P® 15-37.5 mg every morning (2 hours after breakfast).

Renal: Use with *caution*; phentermine is excreted in urine and increases in exposure can be expected.

Hepatic: No adjustment.

Equivalent Dose Phentermine HCl	Equivalent Dose Phentermine Base
8 mg	6.4 mg
15 mg	12 mg
30 mg	24 mg
37.5 mg	30 mg

NON-AMPHETAMINE

Orlistat (Alli™; Xenical®) [19,20]

Available: 60 mg and 120 mg capsules

Dose: *Alli™:* 60 mg TID with each meal containing fat. *Xenical®:* 120 mg TID with each meal containing fat.

Renal: No adjustment

Hepatic: No adjustment

- MOA: Gastrointestinal lipase inhibitor; blocks absorption of dietary fat
- Alli™ is OTC whereas Xenical® is a prescription medication
- Orlistat may reduce the absorption of fat-soluble vitamins A, D, E, K, and beta-carotene. A multivitamin containing these vitamins at least 2 hours before or after orlistat.
- Take during meal or up to 1 hour after meal.
- Steatorrhea/oily anal leakage is a common side effect.

Liraglutide (Saxenda®; Victoza®) [21,22]

Available: 18 mg/3 mL prefilled pen syringe for subcutaneous (SQ) use

Dose: 0.6 mg SQ DAILY for 1 Week then increase by 0.6 mg at weekly intervals until 3 mg/day reached. Discontinue if patient cannot tolerate 3 mg dose as lower doses not proven to be effective.

Renal: Limited experience; use with *caution*

Hepatic: Limited experience; use with *caution*

- MOA: incretin mimetics; glucagon-like peptide-1 (GLP-1) agonist.
- Titration required to reduce GI symptoms.
- If more than 3 days missed, reinitiate at 0.6 mg dose and re-titrate.
- Victoza® approved for adjunct to improve glycemic control in diabetes; whereas, Saxenda® approved for adjunct for chronic weight management.

Lorcaserin (Belviq®; Belviq XR®) [23-25]

Dose: 10 mg BID or 20mg XR daily.

Renal: *CrCl 30-50 mL/min:* use with caution.

CrCl < 30ml/min: not recommended.

Hepatic: *Severe hepatic impairment (Child-Pugh Class C):* use with caution.

- MOA: 5-HT$_{2c}$ receptor agonist (results in satiety & decreased food intake).
- Evaluate response to therapy after 12 weeks; if patient has not lost > 5% baseline body weight then discontinue therapy.

Naltrexone/Bupropion (Contrave®) [25,26]

Dose: Titrate to 32/360 mg per day over the course of 4 weeks as follows:
1 tablet every morning for 7 days → 1 tablet BID for 7 days → 2 tablets every morning & 1 tablet in the evening for 7 days → 2 tablets BID.

Renal: *Moderate to severe*-max dose of 8/90 mg BID. *Severe or ESRD (est GFR of ≤ 20ml/min)*-not recommended.

Hepatic: Impairment-max dose of 8/90 mg per day.

- Evaluate response to therapy after 12 weeks; if patient has not lost > 5% baseline body weight then discontinue therapy
- Max of 8/90mg/day with CYP2B6 Inhibitors (i.e. ticlopidine, clopidogrel)
- As with each individual medication-avoid with eating disorders, seizures, opioid use, MAOI therapy, etc.

Phentermine/Topiramate (Qsymia®) [25,27-30]

Dose: Once daily dosing in the morning with titration required:
3.75/23 mg every morning for 14 days → 7.5/46 mg every morning; evaluate weight loss after 12 weeks. If patient has not lost ≥ 3% of baseline weight, then discontinue therapy OR increase dose to 11.25/69 mg every morning for 14 days → 15/92 mg every morning

Renal: *CrCl < 50 mL/min:* do not exceed 7.5/46 mg per day; *ESRD or dialysis:* AVOID

Hepatic: *Moderate hepatic impairment (Child-Pugh Class B):* 7.5/46 mg/day. *Severe hepatic impairment (Child-Pugh Class C):* avoid use.

- REMS PROGRAM: Qsymia® REMS with only certified pharmacies able to distribute. Available via 1-888-998-4887 or www.QsymiaREMS.com.
- Evaluate weight loss at highest dose after additional 12 weeks; if patient has not lost > 5% baseline body weight then discontinue therapy.
- Discontinue the 15 mg/92 mg dose gradually by dosing every other day for at least 1 week prior to stopping treatment altogether, to avoid precipitating a seizure.
- The 3.75/23 mg and 11.25/69 mg dose are for titration purposes only.
- Early morning dosing preferred; avoid late evening dosing due to insomnia.

For treatment of acquired, generalized hypoactive sexual desire disorder (HSDD) in pre-menopausal women (female sexual interest/arousal disorder):

<u>Flibanserin (Addyi®)</u> [31]

Available: 100 mg tablet

<u>Dose:</u> 100 mg HS and discontinue in 8 weeks if no improvement.

<u>Renal:</u> No adjustment.

<u>Hepatic:</u> *Do not use* in any degree of hepatic impairment.

- MOA: $5\text{-}HT_{1A}$ receptor agonist & $5\text{-}HT_{2A}$ receptor antagonist; additionally, has moderate antagonist activities at the $5\text{-}HT_{2B}$, $5\text{-}HT_{2C}$, and D_4 receptors.
- Pharmacokinetic Information:
  - metabolized via CYP3A4, CYP2C19, P-glycoprotein (P-gp).
  - Inhibits P-gp.
  - Half-life: 11 hours.
- REMS Program: Addyi® REMS program with certified prescribers and dispensing pharmacies at 1-844-746-5745 or visit <u>www.AddyiREMS.com</u>.
- Due to a potential risk for severe hypotension and syncope, especially when combined with alcohol, the product label carries a boxed warning, and a restricted risk evaluation and mitigation strategy (REMS) distribution program has been created for prescribers and dispensing pharmacies. Patients must not use alcohol during treatment.
- **Do not administer with moderate or strong CYP3A4 inhibitors, grapefruit juice and/or EtOH** as may increase risk of severe hypotension or syncope. If initiating Flibanserin after use of moderate/strong CYP3A4 inhibitor wait for 2 weeks after last dose.

For the treatment of pseudobulbar affect (PBA):

<u>Dextromethorphan/Quinidine (Nuedexta®)</u> [32]

Available: 20/10 mg capsule

<u>Dose:</u> 1 capsule (20/10 mg) daily for 7 days → 1 capsule every 12 hours.

<u>Renal:</u> No adjustment; not studied in severe renal impairment.

<u>Hepatic:</u> No adjustment; not studied in severe hepatic impairment.

- MOA: NMDA receptor antagonist & sigma-1 agonist of Dextromethorphan which is inhibited via CYP 2D6 of Quinidine.
- Pharmacokinetic Information:
  - Metabolized via CYP 2D6 & 3A4 and P-gp.
  - Inhibits CYP 2D6.
  - Half-life: 7 hours (Quinidine) & 13 hours (Dextromethorphan).
- PBA occurs secondary to various unrelated neurological conditions and is characterized by uncontrollable, sudden, and frequent episodes of laughing and/or crying.

Alzheimer's Dementia (AD)

Alzheimer's Disease

1. Criteria are met for major or mild neurocognitive disorder.
2. Insidious onset & gradual progression of impairment in one or more cognitive domains (at least two domains for major neurocognitive disorder).
3. Criteria are met for either probable or possible Alzheimer's disease as follows:

   FOR MAJOR NEUROCOGNITIVE DISORDER:

   Probable Alzheimer's disease is diagnosed if either of the following is present; otherwise, **possible Alzheimer's disease** should be diagnosed:

   A. Evidence of a causative Alzheimer's disease genetic mutation from a family history or genetic testing.
   B. All three of the following are present:
      1) Clear evidence of decline in memory and learning and at least one other cognitive domain (based on detailed history or serial neuropsychological testing).
      2) Steadily progressive, gradual decline in cognition, without extended plateaus.
      3) No evidence of mixed etiology (i.e. absence of other neurodegenerative or cerebrovascular disease, or another neurological, mental or systematic disease/condition contributing to cognitive decline).

   FOR MILD NEUROCOGNITIVE DISORDER:

   Probable Alzheimer's disease is diagnosed if there is evidence of a causative Alzheimer's disease genetic mutation from either genetic testing of family history.

   Possible Alzheimer's disease is diagnosed if there is no evidence of a causative Alzheimer's disease genetic mutation from either genetic testing or family history, and all three of the following are present:
      1) Clear evidence of decline in memory and learning.
      2) Steadily progressive, gradual decline in cognition, without extended plateaus.
      3) No evidence of mixed etiology (i.e. absence of other neurodegenerative or cerebrovascular disease, or another neurological or systemic disease/condition likely contributing to cognitive decline).

4. The disturbance is not better explained by cerebrovascular disease, another neurodegenerative disease, the effects of a substance, or another mental, neurological or systemic disorder. [1]

Table 1 describes dosage form, route of administration, and usual daily dose of various medications used for Alzheimer's Disease:

Generic Name	Brand Name	Dosage Form*	Route	Dose Range
Donepezil	Aricept®/ODT™	ODT, L, T	PO	5-23 mg
Galantamine	Razadyne®/ER®	ERC, L, T	PO	4-12 mg BID 8-24 mg ER
Rivastig-mine	Exelon®	C, TP	PO	1.5-6 mg BID 4.6-13.3 mg (24hr patch)
Memantine	Namenda® /XR®	ERT, L, T	PO	5-20 mg IR 7-28 mg ER
Donepezil/ Memantine	Namzaric®	ERC	PO	10/14-10/28 mg

*T: Tablet, L: Liquid for oral use, ERC: Extended-Release Capsule, ERT: Extended-Release Tablet, ODT: oral disintegrating tablets, TP: Transdermal Patch

Table 2 describes various pharmacokinetic profiles of medications used for Alzheimer's Disease, including mechanism of action (MOA), half-life ($t_{1/2}$), and metabolizing/inhibited enzymes:

Drug	MOA[#]	$T_{1/2}$ (Hours)*	Metabolism^	Enzyme Inhibited
Donepezil	AChI	70	CYP 2D6 & 3A4	N/A
Galantamine[H, R]	AChI	7	CYP 2D6 & 3A4	N/A
Rivastigmine[H, R]	AChI	PO: 1.5 Patch: 3[#]	Hydrolysis	N/A
Memantine[H, R]	NMDA Antagonist	60-80	Hydrolysis, glucuronidation	N/A
Donepezil/ Memantine[H, R]	AChI + NMDA Antagonist	60-80	CYP 2D6 & 3A4 Hydrolysis & glucuronidation	N/A

[H]Caution advised in hepatic impairment   [R] Caution advised in renal impairment

*After Oral Administration, [#]AChI: Acetylcholinesterase Inhibitor, NMDA: N-Methyl-D-Aspartate, [#]:(T ½ once removed)

110

Table 3 describes FDA approved indications for various drugs:

Drug	Alzheimer Dementia, mild-moderate	Alzheimer Dementia, moderate-severe	Misc.
Donepezil	X	X (10-23mg)	
Galantamine	X		
Rivastigmine	X	X (patch only)	PDD*
Memantine		X	
Donepezil/ Memantine		X	
*PDD: Parkinson's Disease Dementia			

CLINICAL PEARLS

- Discontinue unnecessary anticholinergic medications [18]
- Precautions with gastrointestinal bleeding and patients with ulcer risks
- Cholinesterase inhibitors (AChI) may have vagotonic effects which may cause bradycardia and/or heart block. Caution in patients at risk of prolonged cardiac repolarization, QT prolongation or torsades de pointes.
- Most common side effect of cholinesterase inhibitors is nausea, vomiting, diarrhea, insomnia, muscle cramps, fatigue and anorexia.
- Low body weight (<50kg) resulted in decrease clearance and may result in increased toxicities and adverse events—consider reducing dose.
- Cognex® (Tacrine) was pulled from market due liver toxicities.[8]

Donepezil (Aricept®/ODT™)[2-3, 17]
Available: 5, 10, 23 mg tablets; 5, 10 mg ODT; 1 mg/ml solution
Dose: **Alzheimer's Disease (AD):** *mild to moderate-* 5 mg QPM x 4-6 weeks → 10 mg QPM, *moderate-severe-* May increase to 23 mg after greater than 3 months of 10 mg/day.
Renal: No adjustment
Hepatic: No adjustment
- Nausea, vomiting and diarrhea are typically transient lasting 1-3 weeks by may persist and appear to be dose related
- Aricept® and Aricept ODT™ are bioequivalent

Galantamine (Razadyne®/ER®)[4-6, 10, 17]

Available: 4, 8, 12mg tablets; 8, 16, 24mg ER capsules; 4mg/ml solution

Dose: **AD:** *mild-moderate:* GIVE WITH MEALS. **IR**: 4mg BID x 4 weeks → 8 mg BID X 4 weeks → 12 mg BID *(as tolerated).* **ER:** 8 mg QAM X 4 weeks → 16 mg QAM X 4 weeks → 24 mg QAM.

Renal: *CrCl of 9-59 mL/min:* max dose of 16 mg/day. *CrCl of < 9 mL/min:* use not recommended

Hepatic: *Moderate impairment (Child-Pugh 7-9):* 16 mg/day. *Severe impairment (Child-Pugh 10-15):* use not recommended

- Conversion from IR tablets and/or solution to ER may be same total dose
- If interrupted for ≥ 3 days, restart at lowest dose & increase to current dose
- Conversion from other AChI may begin immediately upon d/c of previous therapy unless experiencing poor tolerability then allow 7-day washout
- Reminyl® changed to Razadyne® in 2005 due to med errors with Amaryl®

Rivastigmine (Exelon®/Patch®) [7-8, 11, 17]

Available: 1.5, 3, 4.5, 6 mg capsules; 4.6, 9.5, 13.3 mg/24 hr transdermal patch

Dose: **AD:** *mild-moderate:* TAKE WITH MEALS. **PO:** 1.5 mg BID x 2 weeks → increase by 3 mg/day every 2 weeks up to 6 mg BID *(as tolerated),* **Patch:** 4.6 mg/24 hr patch Qdaily; may increase every 4 weeks. *AD, mild-severe:* transdermal only form approved for severe. *Parkinson disease dementia (PDD), mild-moderate:* dose titration above with PO dose increases every 4 weeks rather than every 2 weeks

Renal: No adjustment though clearance may be reduced in moderate to severe renal impairment *(<50 mL/min)* and may need to reduce dose

Hepatic: *Mild-moderate impairment:* clearance reduced may require lower dose; transdermal patch suggest max dose of 4.6 mg/24 hours

- Administer with meals, delays absorption by 90 minutes, may reduce GI adverse events.
- If gastrointestinal adverse events occur discontinue treatment for several doses then restart at same or lower dose
- If stopped for > 3 days restart at 1.5mg BID or 4.6mg/24hr patch
- Patch should be applied to dry, hairless area and changed every 24 hours though upper/lower back preferred as patient less likely to remove
- Remove patch (contains aluminum or other metal components) prior to magnetic resonance imaging (MRI) to avoid overheating & skin burns
- Conversion from Oral to Transdermal:
  < 6mg/day → 4.6mg/24hr patch & 6-12mg/day → 9.5mg/24hr patch

<u>Memantine (Namenda®/XR®)</u>[12-15, 17]

Available: 5, 10 mg tablets; 7, 14, 21, 28 mg ER capsules; 10 mg/5 mL solution

<u>Dose:</u> **AD:** *moderate-severe*: **IR:** 5 mg Qdaily for 1 week → 5 mg BID for 1 week → 5 mg QAM & 10mg bedtime for 1 week → 10 mg BID

ER: 7 mg QDAILY → increase by 7 mg every week up to 28 mg/day

<u>Renal:</u> *CrCl 5-29 mL/min:* no more than IR: 5 mg BID or ER: 14 mg/day

<u>Hepatic:</u> *Severe impairment*: use with caution

- Conversion of IR to ER: 5 mg BID → 14 mg/day or 10 mg BID →28 mg/day
- XR titration packs available

<u>Memantine/Donepezil (Namzaric®)</u>[16]

Available: 7/10, 14/10, 21/10, 28/10 mg ER capsules

<u>Dose:</u> 7/10 mg QPM with dose increases by 7 mg weekly (as tolerated)

<u>Renal:</u> *Severe impairment (CrCl 5-29 mL/min):* 14/10 mg QPM

<u>Hepatic:</u> *Severe impairment*: use with caution

- Patients on Donepezil 10mg only the recommended starting dose is Namzaric® 7/10 mg QPM. If they are on Memantine 10 mg BID or 28 mg ER & Donepezil 10 mg they can be placed on Namzaric® 28/10 mg QPM
- XR titration packs available

Parkinson's Disease (PD)/Restless Legs Syndrome (RLS)/Extrapyramidal Side Effects (EPS)

This section includes:
- A general overview of anticholinergic and anti-parkinson medications
- Classes of medication charts
- Dose form, route and dosage range table
- Pharmacokinetics table
- FDA approved uses
- Clinical pearls

CLINICAL PEARLS

- Levodopa is well-established as the most effective drug for symptomatic treatment of PD and is the drug of first choice
- Dopamine agonists may be used as single drug in early stages of PD or as adjunctive therapy to Carbidopa/Levodopa later in therapy
- Anticholinergics are used as an adjunct in the therapy of all forms of parkinsonism
- COMT Inhibitors are used in PD as adjunctive treatment to Carbidopa/Levodopa
- MAOI-B are used as monotherapy or adjunctive treatment to Carbidopa/Levodopa (with exception of Rasagiline which may be used adjunctively with other Parkinson's Disease medications)
- Amantadine can be used in PD as monotherapy or adjunctive therapy

Dopamine
(DA)

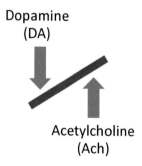

Acetylcholine
(Ach)

Under normal conditions dopamine & acetylcholine are in an electrochemical balance. In Parkinson's there is decreased dopamine in basal ganglia which leads to increased cholinergic sensitivity. Anticholinergics or dopamine agonists will help to improve PD or EPS symptoms.

Table 1 describes dosage form, route of administration, and usual daily dose of various medications used for PD, RLS, and EPS:

Generic Name	Brand Name	Dosage Form*	Route	Dose Range
Amantadine	Symmetrel®	C, L, T	PO	100-400 mg/day
Apomorphine	Apokyn®	SI	SQ	1-20 mg/day
Benztropine	Cogentin®	SI, T	IM, IV, PO	0.5-8 mg/day
Bromocriptine	Parlodel®	C, T	PO	1.25-100 mg/day
Carbidopa	Lodosyn®	T	PO	25-200 mg/day
Carbidopa/ Levodopa	Duopa™ Rytary™ Sinemet®/CR®	ERC, ERT, ODT, S, T	PO; Enteral	See per product in clinical pearls
Carbidopa/ Levodopa/ Entacapone	Stalevo®	T	PO	12.5/50/200 mg - 75/300/400 mg TID
Diphenhy-dramine	Benadryl®	C, Ch, L, ODT, SI, T	IM, IV, PO	IM/IV-10-400 mg/day PO-25-300 mg TID
Entacapone	Comtan®	T	PO	200 mg TID up to 8 times per day
Pramipexole	Mirapex®/ER®	ERT, T	PO	0.125 mg/day – 1.5 mg TID
Generic Name	Brand Name	Dosage Form*	Route	Dose Range
Rasagiline	Azilect®	T	PO	0.5-1 mg/day
Ropinirole	Requip®/ER®	ERT, T	PO	0.25 mg TID–8mg TID
Rotigotine	Neupro®	TP	TP	1-8 mg/24hr
Safinamide	Xadago®	T	PO	50-100 mg/day
Selegiline	Eldepryl® Zelapar®	C, ODT, T	PO	5 mg BID or 1.25-2.5 mg/day (ODT)
Tolcapone	Tasmar®	T	PO	100-200 mg TID
Trihexy-phenidyl	Artane®	L, T	PO	1-15 mg/day
Valbenazine	Ingrezza™	C	PO	80 mg/day

*C: Capsule, Ch: Chewable, L: Liquid for oral use, DRC: Delayed Release Capsule, ERC: Extended-Release Capsule, ERT: Extended-Release Tablet, ODT: Orally Disintegrating Tablet, SI: Solution/suspension for injection, T: Tablet, SL: Sublingual Tablets, TP: Transdermal Patch, S: Suspension for enteral use

Table 2 describes various pharmacokinetic profiles of medications for PD, RLS, & EPS:

Drug	MOA[#]	$T_{1/2}$ (Hours)*	Metabolism^	Enzyme Inhibited
Amantadine[R]	Unknown	11-15	Renal Elimination	N/A
Apomorphine[H,R]	D Agonist	0.5-1	Glucuronidation; Sulfation; N-demethylation	N/A
Benztropine	Ach	1.7-5	N-oxidation; N-dealkylation	N/A
Bromocriptine[H,R]	D Agonist	3-6	CYP 3A4	N/A
Carbidopa	Decarbox Inhibitor	1-2	Renal elimination	N/A
Carbidopa/ Levodopa	See Ind Drugs	1-2	Renal Elimination	N/A
Carbidopa/ Levodopa/ Entacapone[H]	See Ind Drugs	1.3-2.4	COMT; Dopa decarboxylase; Glucuronidation	N/A
Diphenhy-dramine[H]	Ach H$_1$ Antag	2-8	CYPs 2D6, 1A2, 2C9, 2C19	N/A
Entacapone[H]	COMT Inhibitor	1-2	Glucuronidation	N/A
Pramipexole[R]	D Agonist	8	Renal Elimination	N/A
Rasagiline[H]	MOAI (MAO-B)	3	CYP 1A2	N/A
Ropinirole[H,R]	D Agonist	6	CYPA 1A2	N/A
Rotigotine[R]	D Agonist	5-7	Conjugation & N-dealkylation	N/A
Safinamide[H]	MAO-B	20-30	Hydrolytic oxidation; N-dealkylation	Inhibits OCT1
Selegiline	MAO-B	10	CYPs 2B6, 2C9 and 3A4/5	N/A
Tolcapone[H]	COMT Inhibitor	2-3	Glucuronidation	N/A
Trihexyphenidyl	Ach	3.7	Renal Elimination	N/A
Valbenazine[R,H]	Reversible VMAT 2 inhibitor	15-22	Hydrolysis &oxidation; CYPs 3A4/5,2D6	N/A

[H] caution advised in hepatic impairment [R] caution advised in renal impairment
*After Oral Administration, #Ach: Anticholinergic, COMT: Catecholamine-O-Methyltransferase, MAOI-Monoamine Oxidase Inhibitor, D Agonist: Dopamine Agonist, Decarbox: Decarboxylase, VMAT: Vesicular Monoamine Transporter 2
^CYP: Cytochrome, UGT-G: UDP-glucuronosyltransferase-Glucuronidation

Table 3 describes various FDA approved indications for drugs used for Parkinson's Disease (PD), Restless Legs Syndrome (RLS), and Extrapyramidal Side Effects (EPS):

	PD*	EPS	RLS	Miscellaneous
Amantadine	X or X^2	X		Influenza
Apomorphine	X^1			
Benztropine	X^2	X		
Bromocriptine	X or X^3			Multiple indications
Carbidopa	X			
Carbidopa/ Levodopa	X			
Carbidopa/ Levodopa/ Entacapone	X			
Diphenhy- dramine	X^2	X		Multiple indications
Entacapone	X^3			
Pramipexole	X or X^3		X	
Rasagiline	X or X^2			
Ropinirole	X or X^3		X	
Rotigotine	X		X	
Safinamide	X^3			
Selegiline	X or X^3			
Tolcapone	X^3			
Trihexyphenidyl	X^2	X		
Valbenazine				Tardive Dyskinesia

*X^1: Advanced Parkinson's Disease for "rescue" in patient with intractable "off" periods; X^2: Adjunct in all forms of Parkinson's Disease; X^3 :Adjunct with Carbidopa/Levodopa

LEVODOPA (L-DOPA) AGENTS:

MOA: Levodopa serves as the precursor for dopamine and converted to dopamine in CNS. Carbidopa is a noncompetitive decarboxylase inhibitor that inhibits peripheral conversion of levodopa to dopamine and increasing CNS bioavailability of levodopa.

Adverse Effects: Dizziness, headache, nausea, somnolence are most common. More serious side effects may include agitation, confusion, delusions, hallucinations, orthostatic hypotension and psychosis. Dyskinesias may occur in long-term therapy (3-5 years)

Contraindications: Closed-angle glaucoma, melanoma (or history of as may activate) and non-selective MAOIs or hypersensitivity to Carbidopa, Levodopa or other component of drug.

Carbidopa/Levodopa (Duopa™; Rytary™; SINEMET®/CR®) [1-4]
Available: 10-100, 25-100, 25-250 mg orally disintegrating tablets;
10-100, 25-100, 25-250 mg tablets; 25-100, 50-200 mg extended-release tablets;
Duopa™: 4.63/20 mg/mL enteral suspension; Rytary™: 23.75-95, 36.25-145,
48.75-195, 61.25-245 mg extended release capsules

Dose: AS FOLLOWS PER SPECIFIC PRODUCT:

IR tablets: 10/100-25/100 mg TID with dose increase of 1 tablet every day to every other day. **CR tablets:** 50/200 mg BID with increase Q3 days as needed (separate dose by 4-8 hours). **Rytary™:** 23.75/95 mg TID x 3D → 36.25/145mg TID (may further titrate based upon response & tolerability). **Duopa™:** *SEE PACKAGE INSERT FOR CALCULATION & PUMP DIRECTIONS*

Max Dose: 10/100 mg tablet is 80/800 mg/day (8 tablets)
                     25/100 mg tablet is 200/800 mg/day (8 tablets)
                     25/250 mg tablet is 200/2000 mg/day (8 tablets)
                     Sinemet CR®: most pts controlled up to 1600 mg/day L-dopa
                     Rytary™: 612.5/2450 mg/day
                     Duopa™: 2000 mg/day of levodopa administered over 16 hours

Renal: No adjustment
Hepatic: No adjustment

- Combination Carbidopa-Levodopa products are marketed in 1:10 or 1:4 ratios; respectively. The addition of Carbidopa allows for lower doses of Levodopa to be used thus which correlates with reducing dopaminergic side effects such as nausea/vomiting.
- Best to take IR version 30-60 mins before meal as protein may interfere with absorption
- At least 70-100mg Carbidopa should be provided per day
- Converting IR to ER tablets—use 10 up to 30% more Levodopa per day

Total Daily Dose of Levodopa in Carbidopa/Levodopa IR	Total Daily Dose of Levodopa in Rytary™
400-549 mg	855 mg ÷ TID
550-749 mg	1140 mg ÷ TID
750-949 mg	1305 mg ÷ TID
950-1249 mg	1705 mg ÷ TID
≥ 1250 mg	2205-2340 mg ÷ TID

Carbidopa/Levodopa/Entacapone (Stalevo®) [5]
Available: 12.5/50/200; 18.75/75/200; 25/100/200; 31.25/125/200;
37.5/150/200; 50/200/200 mg tablets

Dose: Direct switch with equivalent individual dosing OR Entacapone naïve patients experiencing signs and symptoms of end-of-dose or "wear off" effect and taking a total daily dose of 600 mg of Levodopa are usually initiated on Entacapone 200mg with each Carbidopa/Levodopa dose & usually a 25% reduction of Levodopa is required (best to add Entacapone as adjuvant first then do a direct switch for tolerance purposes)

Max dose: 8 tablets of Stalevo® (50-,75-,100-,125-,150 mg of Levodopa) and 6 tablets of Stalevo® (200 mg of Levodopa)

Renal: No adjustment

Hepatic: *Caution* advised; AUC & Cmax of Entacapone increase in impairment.

- Each tablet contains 200 mg of Entacapone
- Max dose of Entacapone is 1600 mg/day

Carbidopa (Lodosyn®) [6]

Available: 25 mg tablets

Dose: 25 mg initial dose with addition of 12.5-25 mg per dose as needed

Max dose of 200 mg/day total carbidopa

Renal: No adjustment

Hepatic: No adjustment

- **Does not cross blood brain barrier (BBB); must always be administered with Levodopa**
- Increases bioavailability of levodopa by inhibiting metabolism of levodopa in GI tract & reduces nausea caused by levodopa alone[3]

DOPAMINE AGONISTS:

MOA: Agonist at dopamine receptors. Ergots (Bromocriptine) not used as commonly as the non-ergots (Apomorphine, Pramipexole, Ropinirole and Rotigotine)

Adverse Effects: Compulsive behaviors (uncontrolled shopping, gambling, eating and sexual urges,) delusions, dyskinesia, hallucinations, hypotension, impulse control, psychosis, somnolence or sleep attacks

Contraindications: Ergot alkaloid hypersensitivity (choose non-ergot) or known hypersensitivity to particular product

Apomorphine (Apokyn®) [7]

Available: 10 mg/mL injections (subcutaneous)

Dose: 2 mg (0.2 mL) SQ as test dose with BP monitoring-if tolerated and response may begin to increase by 1 mg (0.1 mL) every few days. If tolerated but no response, see PI for further testing/titration instructions

Max dose: 0.6 mL (6 mg) per injection; max of 5 injections/day not to exceed 2 mL (20 mg/day)

Renal: Starting dose for *mild-mod impairment* should be 1 mg (0.1 mL)

Hepatic: *Caution* in hepatic impairment; moderate impairment may result in increased AUC (10%) & Cmax (25%)

- Indicated as acute/intermittent treatment of hypomobility or rescue of "off" or "end-of-dose wearing off" episodes with advanced Parkinson's

- Strong emetic effect; therefore, recommend to provide with antiemetic 3 days before use though not 5HT3 antagonists (*contraindicated*)
- BP must be monitored (pre-dose, 20, 40 and 60 minutes' post dose)
- Contains sodium metabisulfite that may cause allergic-type reactions in those with sulfite sensitivity.

Bromocriptine (Parlodel®) [8]
Available: 2.5 mg tablets; 5 mg capsules
Dose: 1.25 mg BID; increase by 2.5 mg/day every 14-28 days
Max dose: 100 mg/day
Renal: *Caution* in renal impairment
Hepatic: *Caution* in hepatic impairment; ergot toxicity potential
- Other indications are Acromegaly and Hyperprolactinemia associated dysfunctions
- Ergoline compound derived from ergot alkaloids—more severe side effects like pulmonary fibrosis. Previous Pergolide (Permax®) was pulled from the market due to pulmonary fibrosis and valvular heart disease.
- Approximate dose equivalency—Bromocriptine to Ropinirole (10:6) and Bromocriptine to Pramipexole (10:1-1.5) [29]

Pramipexole (Mirapex®/ER®) [9-10]
Available: 0.125, 0.25, 0.5, 0.75, 1 and 1.5 mg tablets; 0.375, 0.75, 1.5, 2.25, 3, 3.75 and 4 mg extended release tablets
Dose: **Parkinson's Disease Dose Titration:**

Week 1	Week 2	Week 3	Week 4	Week 5	Week 6	Week 7
0.125 mg TID	0.25 mg TID	0.5 mg TID	0.75 mg TID	1 mg TID	1.25 mg TID	1.5 mg TID

Restless Legs Syndrome Dose Titration:

Step 1	Step 2 (if needed)	Step 3 (if needed)
0.125 mg	0.25 mg	0.5 mg
4-7 days	4-7 days	4-7 days

Renal:
  Immediate Release:
  CrCl 35-59 mL/min: 0.125 mg BID initially; max of 1.5 mg BID
  CrCl 15-34 mL/min: 0.125mg Qdaily; max of 1.5 mg daily
  CrCl < 15 mL/min: not adequately studied
  Extended-release:
  CrCl 30-50 mL/min: 0.375 mg every other day; titrate by 0.375 mg increments at a minimum of weekly intervals; max of 2.25mg/day
  CrCl < 30mL/min: not recommended
Hepatic: No adjustment

Ropinirole (Requip®/XL®) [11-12]

Available: 0.25, 0.5, 1, 2, 3, 4, 5 mg tablets; 2, 4, 6, 8, 12 mg ER tablets

Dose: **Parkinson's Disease Dose Titration:**

Week 1	Week 2	Week 3	Week 4
0.25 mg TID	0.5 mg TID	0.75 mg TID	1 mg TID
After Week 4 may increase by 1.5mg/day up to 9mg/day			
Then by 3mg/day up to Max of 24mg/day			

RLS Dose Titration:

Days 1-2	Days 3-7	Week 2	Week 3	Week 4	Week 5	Week 6	Week 7
0.25 mg	0.5 mg	1 mg	1.5 mg	2 mg	2.5 mg	3 mg	4 mg

Renal: *CrCl < 15mL/min* & receiving hemodialysis with reduced max dose of 18 mg/day for PD and 3 mg/day in RLS

Hepatic: Titrate initial dose with caution

- Discontinuation—taper gradually over 7-day period.
- Convert IR to ER/XL as follows:

Immediate-Release Ropinirole Tablets (TDD-total daily dose in mg)								
0.75-2.25	3-4	6	7.5-9	12	15	18	21	24
Extended-Release Ropinirole Tablets (TDD-total daily dose in mg)								
2	4	6	8	12	16	18	20	24

Rotigotine (Neupro®) [13-14]

Available: 1, 2, 3, 4, 6 and 8 mg/24-hour transdermal patch

Dose: **PD:** 2 mg/24hr for early-stage PD and 4 mg/24hr for advanced-stage PD. The dose may be increased by 2 mg/24hr once weekly up to 6 mg/24hr in early-stage and 8 mg/24hr in advanced-stage. *RLS:* 1 mg/24hr increased by 1 mg/24hr once weekly up to 3 mg/24hr

Renal: No adjustment; though exposure to rotigotine conjugates was doubled in severe impairment (*15-29 mL/min*)

Hepatic: No adjustment

- Apply patch to clean, dry and healthy skin on the stomach, thigh, hip, side of body between ribs and pelvis (flank), shoulder or upper arm.
- Patch should not be applied to same area more than once per 14 days.
- Contains sodium metabisulfite that may cause allergic-type reactions in those with sulfite sensitivity.
- For moderate to severe RLS
- Remove patch before defibrillation (cardioversion) or MRI.
- For discontinuation reduce by 2 mg/24hr every other day in PD and 1 mg/24hr every other day in RLS.

ANTICHOLINERGICS:

<u>MOA</u>: Compete with acetylcholine (Ach) at muscarinic receptors in the CNS. Can block reuptake of dopamine in CNS thus prolonging dopamine's effect.

<u>Adverse Effects</u>: Anticholinergic effects (blurred vision, cognitive impairment, constipation, urinary retention, xerostomia, etc.), dizziness, drowsiness, mydriasis, tachycardia.

<u>Contraindications</u>: Closed-angle glaucoma, caution in asthma & COPD, caution in bladder obstruction, GI obstruction, benign prostatic hypertrophy and/or urinary retention, caution in geriatric patients

> **ANTI-SLUDGE:**
> Salivation
> Lacrimation
> Urination
> Defecation
> GI irritation
> Eye constriction

<u>Benztropine (Cogentin®)</u> [15-17]

Available: 0.5, 1 and 2 mg tablets; 1 mg/1 mL solution for injection
<u>Dose:</u> **PD:** 0.5-1 mg PO or IM HS may increase by 0.5 mg every 5-6 days. **EPS:** 1-4 mg PO, IM or IV BID; typical dose 1-2 mg BID-TID. Max dose: 8 mg/day
<u>Renal:</u> No adjustment
<u>Hepatic:</u> No adjustment

- Tertiary amine, crosses blood brain barrier (BBB) into CNS, but less CNS stimulation than Trihexyphenidyl
- Cumulative effect and may take 2-3 days for therapeutic effect
- Longer duration and may require less frequent dosing than Diphenhydramine
- Acute dystonic reactions typically respond to 1-2 mg IM or IV followed by oral dose to prevent recurrence

<u>Diphenhydramine (Benadryl®)</u> [18-19]

Available: 12.5 mg chewable tablets; 12.5 mg/5 mL oral solution; 12.5, 25 mg ODT and dissolving film; 25, 50 mg capsule; 25, 50 mg tablet; 50 mg/1mL solution for injection
<u>Dose:</u> **PD:** 25 mg TID may increase to 50 mg QID. **PD or EPS**: 10-50mg IM/IV
<u>Max Dose:</u> 300 mg/day PO; 400 mg/day IM/IV
<u>Renal:</u> No adjustment
<u>Hepatic:</u> Dose reduction may be warranted; extensively metabolized

- Onset of EPS action with IM is typically 15-30 minutes
- Onset of PO action is 15-30 minutes with peak of 2-4 hours

<u>Trihexyphenidyl (Artane®)</u> [20]

Available: 2 mg/5 mL Oral Elixir & Oral Solution; 2 and 5 mg tablets
<u>Dose:</u> **PD:** 1 mg initially; may increase to 2mg after 3-5 days until 6-10mg/day reached; some patients may require dose of 12-15 mg/day. Usually given as TID-QID with meals and/or at bedtime. **EPS:** 1 mg initially; may repeat in several hours; increase to range of 5 to 15 mg per day

Max dose: 15 mg/day
Renal: No adjustment
Hepatic: No adjustment
- Tertiary antimuscarinic with actions similar to atropine. Since it's a tertiary compound it will penetrate CNS making it useful in Parkinson's.

COMT INHIBITORS:

MOA: Selective inhibitor of peripheral catechol-O-methyltransferase (COMT) which acts to eliminate biologically active catechols and their metabolites. (Prolongs plasma T ½ of levodopa & increases duration of action thus decreasing the daily levodopa requirements.)
Adverse Effects: Dyskinesias/hyperkinesis/hypokinesis, diarrhea, dizziness, drowsiness, nausea, urine discoloration
Contraindications: Hypersensitivity to known particular product; hepatic disease or history of rhabdomyolysis in Tolcapone

Entacapone (Comtan®) [21]
Available: 200 mg tablet
Dose: 200 mg with each dose of Carbidopa/Levodopa up 8 times per day
Max Dose: 1600 mg/day
Renal: No adjustment
Hepatic: *Caution* advised; AUC & Cmax of Entacapone increase in impairment
- Majority of patients will require 25% reduction of daily Levodopa dose
- Adjuvant to Carbidopa/Levodopa for end-of-dose "wear off" effect

Tolcapone (Tasmar®) [22]
Available: 100 and 200 mg tablets
Dose: 100 mg TID; may increase to 200 mg TID
Renal: *Mild-mod impairment (CrCl > 25 mL/min)* no adjustments
CrCl < 25 mL/min not studied; not expected to be removed by HD
Hepatic: **DISCONTINUE** if LFTs exceed 2 times upper limits of normal
- Black box warning of hepatotoxicity—recommended to monitor LFTs at baseline, then periodically (every 2-4 weeks) for first 6 months and then periodically as deemed clinically relevant.
- If no benefit after 3 weeks Tolcapone should be discontinued.

MOA-B INHIBITORS:

MOA: Irreversible inhibitor of monoamine oxidase (MAO) enzyme system. Serotonin and norepinephrine are primarily metabolized via MAO-A whereas dopamine is metabolized via MAO-B. Inhibitory action specific to MAO-B results in increased extracellular levels of dopamine.
Adverse Effects: Anxiety, ataxia, dizziness, dyskinesia, hallucinations, headache, hypertension, insomnia, nausea, orthostatic hypotension

Contraindications: Cyclobenzaprine, Dextromethorphan, Meperidine, Methadone, St. John's Wort and Tramadol or receiving any other MAOI therapy, pheochromocytoma, or hypersensitivity to know particular product.

Rasagiline (Azilect®) [23]
Available: 0.5 and 1 mg tablets
<u>Dose:</u> Adjunctive therapy: 0.5 mg daily; may increase to 1 mg daily
Monotherapy or adjunct (not taking L-dopa): 1 mg daily
<u>Max Dose:</u> 1 mg/day due to risk of hypertension
<u>Renal:</u> No adjustment
<u>Hepatic:</u> *Mild impairment-* Do not exceed 0.5 mg daily. Should not use in moderate/severe impairment

- When used with **CYP1A2 inhibitors** require dose adjustment & lower max dose (0.5 mg/day) as concentrations of Rasagiline expected to double
- Recommended to avoid use with other serotonergic medications
- Dietary restrictions not required (foods high in tyramine ≥ 150 mg i.e. Stilton age cheese should be avoided)

Safinamide (Xadago®) [30]
Available: 50 and 100 mg tablets
<u>Dose:</u> Adjunctive therapy: 50 mg daily; may increase to 100 mg daily
<u>Max Dose:</u> 100 mg/day
<u>Renal:</u> No adjustment
<u>Hepatic:</u> *Moderate impairment (Child-Pugh 7-9):* lower dose of 50 mg/day. *Severe impairment (Child-Pugh 10-15):* contraindicated

- Additionally inhibits release of glutamate, blocks Na & Ca channels and inhibits Dopamine reuptake.
- Concomitant use with Fluoxetine or Fluvoxamine should be avoided; otherwise, use lowest possible doses.
- Do no administer to patients with ophthalmological history at risk for potential retinal effects (i.e. albino patients, family history of hereditary retinal disease, retinitis pigmentosa, active retinopathy or uveitis)
- Common possible side effects are falls, nausea, insomnia, dyskinesia (most common,) somnolence, dizziness, headache, cataract and orthostatic hypotension

Selegiline (Eldepryl®; Zelapar®) [24-25]
Available: 1.25 mg orally disintegrating tablets & 5 mg capsules/tablets
<u>Dose:</u> *Tablets/Capsules*: 5 mg BID (breakfast & lunch)
  ODT: 1.25 mg QAM (breakfast-avoid food/liquid 5 mins before/after.) May increase to 2.5 mg after 6 weeks (higher doses have not shown added benefit or been established).
<u>Renal:</u> No adjustment

<u>Hepatic:</u> No adjustment
- Metabolized to L-methamphetamine & L-amphetamine
- No dietary restrictions if dose is ≤ 10 mg/day (presumably selective inhibits MOA-B)
- Risks for phenylketonuric patients as each ODT contains 1.25 mg of phenylalanine (a component of aspartame.)

<u>MISCELLANEOUS:</u>

<u>MOA:</u> Not fully understood though thought to potentiate CNS dopaminergic response by increasing dopamine release and decreasing dopamine re-uptake into presynaptic neurons. Helps to restore balance of Ach & DA.
<u>Adverse Effects:</u> Dizziness, insomnia most common; less frequent-anxiety, ataxia, confusion, depression, drowsiness, hallucinations, headache, irritability, nervousness and nightmares
<u>Contraindications:</u> Amantadine or Rimantadine hypersensitivity

<u>Amantadine (Symmetrel®)</u> [26-28]
Available: 100 mg capsules; 100mg tablets; 50mg/5ml oral solution
<u>Dose:</u> Monotherapy: 100 mg BID with Max dose of 400 mg/day
Other antiparkinsonian meds: 100 mg daily for 7 days then 100 mg BID
<u>Renal:</u> *CrCl 30-50 mL/min:* 200 mg for 1st day; reduce to 100 mg/day. *CrCl 15-29 mL/min:* 100 mg for 1st day; reduce to 100 mg every other day. *CrCl < 15mL/min:* reduce dose and interval to 200 mg every 7 days
<u>Hepatic:</u> *Caution* recommended; dose adjustment unnecessary
- Crosses blood brain barrier (BBB) and less effective than levodopa
- Offers additional benefit in patients experiencing maximal or waning effects from levodopa
- Indicated for Parkinson's and EPS (also influenza)
- Acidifying urine increases rate of excretion

For the treatment of chorea associated with Huntington's Disease:
<u>Tetrabenazine (Xenazine®)</u> [32,33]
Available: 12.5 and 25 mg tablets
<u>Dose:</u> 12.5 mg every morning for 7 days → 12.5 mg BID; may be further increased by 12.5 mg/day each week as tolerated to reduce chorea. Max single dose is 25 mg and doses above this should be administered in divided doses. Max dose of 100 mg/day for CYP2D6 extensive or intermediate metabolizers, or 50 mg/day for CYP2D6 poor metabolizers.
<u>Renal:</u> No adjustment.
<u>Hepatic:</u> *Contraindicated* in hepatic impairment.
- MOA: Inhibitor of vesicular monoamine transporter 2 (VMAT2) resulting in decreased uptake of monoamines into synaptic vesicles and depletion of monoamine stores (selective, reversible, centrally-acting dopamine

depletor-depletes presynaptic dopamine, norepinephrine and serotonin storage and antagonizes postsynaptic dopamine receptors).
- Pharmacokinetic Information:
  - Extensively hepatically metabolized and renally eliminated
  - Half-life: 7-12 hours.
- Monitor for worsening depression, suicidality or unusual changes in behavior. Tetrabenazine causes QT prolongation of ~ 8msec.
- Physician and patient must complete and sign Xenazine® Treatment Form and faxed to Xenazine® Information Center at 1-888-882-6013 and filled via a Specialty Pharmacy.
- May be discontinued without tapering dose. Treatment interruption of > 5 days requires re-titration.

For the Treatment of Tardive Dyskinesia:

Valbenazine (Ingrezza ™) [31]
Available: 40 mg capsules
Dose: 40 mg daily for 7 days, then 80 mg daily.
Renal: *Not recommended* in severe renal impairment (*CrCl <30 mL/min*)
Hepatic: *Moderate-severe impairment (Child-Pugh 7-15):* 40 mg/day

- MOA: Reversible inhibitor of vesicular monoamine transporter 2 (VMAT2)
- Undergoes hepatic metabolism by hydrolysis and oxidative metabolism, primarily CYPs 3A4 and 3A5 and further metabolized in part by CYP2D6 with some renal elimination.
- Monitor for somnolence and caution with QT prolongation (more so a concern if patient is taking strong CYP2D6 or CYP3A4 inhibitor.

Dose Adjustments via Drug Interactions:

Factors	Dose Adjustments for INGREZZA™
Use of MAOIs	Avoid concomitant use with MAOIs
Use of Strong CYP3A4 Inducers	Concomitant use is not recommended
Use of Strong CYP3A4 Inhibitors	Reduce dose to 40mg
Use of Strong CYP2D6 Inhibitors	Consider dose reduction based on tolerability

Free Resourceful Websites

DailyMed (Package Inserts): https://dailymed.nlm.nih.gov/dailymed/index.cfm

CenterWatch (New FDA approvals per therapeutic area):
https://www.centerwatch.com/drug-information/fda-approved-drugs/therapeutic-areas

FDA (Recalls, MedWatch, Safety Alerts, News and Events):
http://www.fda.gov/

FDA Advisory Committee Reports (FDA labels, approval and Advisory Committee reports):
http://www.accessdata.fda.gov/scripts/cder/drugsatfda/

FDA Shortages (Drug Shortages):
http://www.accessdata.fda.gov/scripts/drugshortages/default.cfm

ASHP Drug Shortages (Drug Shortages):
http://www.ashp.org/shortages

Orange Book (Approved Therapeutic Equivalence):
http://www.accessdata.fda.gov/scripts/cder/ob/default.cfm

Pillbox (Rapid Pill Identification):
https://pillbox.nlm.nih.gov/pillimage/search.php

National Guidelines (Current treatment guidelines):
https://www.guidelines.gov/

DEA Regulations Practitioners Per State:
https://www.deadiversion.usdoj.gov/drugreg/practioners/mlp_by_state.pdf

Drug Patent Expirations:
http://www.uspto.gov/patent/laws-and-regulations/patent-term-extension/patent-terms-extended-under-35-usc-156

USP Verified Supplements:
http://www.quality-supplements.org/

GlobalRph (Clinician's Guide—Kinetics, Calculators, Medication Tables, Etc.):
http://www.globalrph.com/

NAMI (National Alliance on Mental Illness) Locate Support Centers, Fact Sheets, Helplines, Etc: http://www.nami.org/#

SAMHSA (Substance Abuse and Mental Health Services Administration) National Suicide Prevention Lifeline, Behavioral Health Treatment Locator, Buprenorphine Physician Locator, Publications, Etc: www.samhsa.gov

Literature Search and Clinical Trial Information:

PubMed (Literature Search):
http://www.ncbi.nlm.nih.gov/pubmed/

ClinicalTrials (Clinical Trials):
https://clinicaltrials.gov/

Pregnancy and Lactation References:

LactMed (Drugs and Lactation Database):
https://toxnet.nlm.nih.gov/newtoxnet/lactmed.htm

MotherToBaby (Fact Sheets Regarding Exposures During Pregnancy and Lactation):
http://mothertobaby.org/fact-sheets-parent/

References

Pharmacokinetics and Bioequivalence

1. *PHARMACIST'S LETTER / PRESCRIBER'S LETTER* February 2007 ~ Volume 23 ~ Number 230201 Active Metabolites: Follow-on Drugs: Therapeutic Benefit or Economic Burden?
2. Sidney H. Kennedy, Henning F. Andersen, and Raymond W. Lam. "Efficacy of escitalopram in the treatment of major depressive disorder compared with conventional selective serotonin reuptake inhibitors and venlafaxine XR: a meta-analysis." J Psychiatry Neurosci. 2006 March; 31(2): 122–131.
3. S. Svensson and P. R. Mansfield. "Escitalopram: superior to citalopram or a chiral chimera?" Psychother Psychosom. 2004 Jan-Feb;73(1):10-6. S. K. Teo et al. "Clinical pharmacokinetics of thalidomide." Clin Pharmacokinet. 2004;43(5):311-27.

Anxiolytics & Hypnotics: (Benzodiazepines, "Z" drugs, Miscellaneous)

1. Michelini S, Cassano GB, Frare F, Perugi G. Long-term use of benzodiazepines: tolerance, dependence and clinical problems in anxiety and mood disorders. Pharmacopsychiatry. 1996;29(4):127-134.
2. Xanax® (alprazolam) package insert. Kalamazoo, MI: Pharmacia & Upjohn Company; 2003 Jan.
3. Xanax (alprazolam) package insert. New York, NY: Pharmacia & Upjohn Company; 2013 Sept.
4. Xanax® XR (alprazolam extended release) package insert. Kalamazoo, MI: Pharmacia & Upjohn Company; 2004 April.
5. Alprazolam orally disintegrating tablets (ODT) package insert. Chestnut Ridge, NY: Par Pharmaceutical; 2016 Sept.
6. Librium (chlordiazepoxide) package insert. Costa Mesa, CA; Valeant Pharmaceuticals International: 2005 Jul.
7. Onfi (clobazam tablets) package insert. Deerfield, IL: Lundbeck Inc.; 2014 Dec.
8. Klonopin® (clonazepam) package insert. Nutley, NJ: Roche Laboratories, Inc; 2016 Mar.
9. Klonopin (clonazepam) package insert. South San Francisco, CA; Genetech, Inc.; 2016 Mar.
10. Tranxene (clorazepate) package insert. Deerfield, IL; Lundbeck Inc.; 2010 May.
11. Valium® (diazepam) package insert. Nutley, NJ: Roche Laboratories, Inc.; 2008 Jan.
12. Diazepam injection package insert. Deerfield, IL: Baxter Healthcare Inc.; 2006 Feb.
13. Diazepam injection package insert. Lake Forest, IL: Hospira, Inc.; 2008 Jan.
14. Diastat (diazepam) package insert. Aliso Viejo, CA: Valeant Pharmaceuticals International; 2014 Dec.
15. Prosom(TM) (estazolam) tablets package insert. North Chicago, IL: Abbott Laboratories; 2004 Jan.
16. Dalmane (flurazepam) package insert. Aliso Viejo, CA: Valeant Pharmaceuticals, International; 2007 Oct.
17. Dalmane® (flurazepam) package insert. Humacao, Puerto Rico: Roche Products, Inc.; 2000 Nov.
18. Ativan (lorazepam) tablets package insert. Bridgewater, NJ: Valeant Pharmaceuticals North American LLC; 2016 Sept.
19. Ativan (lorazepam) injection package insert. Eatontown, NJ: West-Ward Pharmaceuticals; 2016 Apr.
20. Ativan (lorazepam) oral concentrate package insert. Amityville, NY: Hi-Tech Pharmacal Co., Inc. 2010 Feb.
21. Versed® (midazolam) package insert. Nutley, NJ: Roche Laboratories, Inc.; 1998 Dec.
22. Oxazepam package insert. Miami, Fl: Ivax Pharmaceuticals, Inc.; 2004 Aug.
23. Doral (quazepam) package insert. Union City, CA: Questcor Pharmaceuticals, Inc.; 2010 Oct.
24. Restoril (temazepam) package insert. Hazelwood, MO: Mallinckrodt, Inc.; 2009 Jun.
25. Halcion (triazolam) package insert. New York, NY: Pharmacia and Upjohn Company; 2014 Sept.
26. Lunesta (eszopiclone) package insert. Marlborough, MA: Sunovion Pharmaceuticals Inc; 2014 May.
27. Sonata (zaleplon) package insert. Bristol, TN: King Pharmaceuticals; 2016 Nov.
28. Ambien CR (zolpidem extended-release tablets) package insert. New York, NY: Sanofi-Synthelabo Inc; 2016 Aug.
29. Intermezzo (zolpidem tartrate) sublingual tablets package insert. Pt. Richmond, CA: Transcept Pharmaceuticals, Inc.; 2015 Sept.
30. Edluar (zolpidem tartrate sublingual tablets) package insert. Somerset NJ: Meda Pharmaceuticals Inc.; 2013 Apr.
31. Zolpimist (zolpidem tartrate) Oral Spray package insert. Richmond, VA: ECR Pharmaceuticals; 2013 Apr.
32. Food and Drug Administration (FDA) Drug Safety Communication: risk of next-morning impairment after use of insomnia drugs; FDA requires lower recommended doses for certain drugs containing zolpidem (Ambien, Ambien CR, Edluar, and Zolpimist). Retrieved January 10, 2013. Available at http://www.fda.gov.lp.hscl.ufl.edu/Drugs/DrugSafety/ucm334033.htm.
33. Ambien (zolpidem immediate-release tablets) package insert. New York, NY: Sanofi-Synthelabo Inc; 2016 Aug.
34. Belsomra (suvorexant) tablets package insert. Whitehouse Station, NJ: Merck Sharp & Dohme Corp.; 2016 Jun.
35. Buspar (buspirone) package insert. Princeton, NJ: Bristol-Myers Squibb Company; 2003 Nov.
36. Vistaril (hydroxyzine hydrochloride) package insert. New York, NY: Pfizer Roerig; 2010 Jun.
37. Vistaril (hydroxyzine pamoate) package insert. New York, NY: Pfizer Labs; 2016 Nov.
38. Atarax (hydroxyzine) tablets and syrup package insert. New York, NY: Pfizer Roerig; 2001.
39. Rozerem (ramelteon) package insert. Lincolnshire, IL: Takeda Pharmaceuticals; 2010 Nov.
40. Flumazenil package insert. Irvine, CA: Sicor Pharmaceuticals Inc.; 2005 Jun.
41. Kato K, Hirai K, Nishiyama K, et al. Neurochemical properties of ramelteon (TAK-375), a selective MT1/MT2 receptor agonist. Neuropharmacology 2005;48:301-10.
42. Food and Drug Administration (FDA). FDA Drug Safety Communication: FDA warns about serious risks and death when combining opioid pain or cough medicines with benzodiazepines; requires its strongest warning. http://www.fda.gov.lp.hscl.ufl.edu/Drugs/DrugSafety/ucm518473.htm. Retrieved August 31, 2016.

43. VA/DoD CLINICAL PRACTICE GUIDELINE FOR THE MANAGEMENT OF SUBSTANCE USE DISORDERS. December 2015 p.90. Available at http://www.healthquality.va.gov/guidelines/MH/sud/VADoDSUDCPGRevised22216.pdf
44. Mendelson WB. A review of the evidence for the efficacy and safety of trazodone in insomnia. J Clin Psychiatry. 2005;66:469-76.
45. Cardinali DP, Srinivasan V, Brzezinski A, et al. Melatonin and its analogs in insomnia and depression. J Pineal Res 2012;52:365-75.
46. Volz HP, Kieser M. Kava-kava extract WS 1490 versus placebo in anxiety disorders--a randomized placebo-controlled 25-week outpatient trial. Pharmacopsychiatry 1997;30:1-5.
47. Health Care Financing Administration. Interpretive Guidelines for Long-term Care Facilities. Title 42 CFR 483.25(l) F329: Unnecessary Drugs. Revised 2015.
48. Bailey L, Ward M, Musa MN. Clinical pharmacokinetics of benzodiazepines. J Clin Pharmacol 1994;34:804-811.
49. Ravindran LN, Stein MB. The pharmacologic treatment of anxiety disorders: a review of progress. J Clin Psychiatry. 2010;71(7):839-854.
50. American Geriatrics Society updated Beers Criteria for potentially inappropriate medication use in older adults. J Am Geriatr Soc. 2012;60(4):616-631.
51. Journal of Clinical Sleep Medicine, Vol. 13, No. 2, 2017 Available at http://www.aasmnet.org/Resources/pdf/PharmacologicTreatmentofInsomnia.pdf
52. Neubauer DN. New and emerging pharmacotherapeutic approaches for insomnia. Int Rev Psychiatry. 2014;26(2):214-224. Doi:10.3109/09540261.2014.88890.
53. Sonka K, Sos P, Susta M. Past and present in drug treatment of sleep disorders. Neuro Endocrinol Lett. 2014;35(3):186-197.
54. Cunnington D, Junge MF, Fernando AT. Insomnia: prevalence, consequences and effective treatment. Med J Aust. 2013;199(8):S36-S40.
55. Ioachimescu OC, El-Solh AA. Pharmacotherapy of insomnia. Expert Opin Pharmacother. 2012; 13(9):1243-1260. Doi:10.1517/14656566.2012.683860.
56. *Hartley LR, Ungapen S, Davie I, Spencer DJ. The effect of beta adrenergic blocking drugs on speakers' performance and memory. Br J Psychiatry. 1983;142:512-517.*

Antidepressants
1. American Psychiatric Association: Diagnostic and Statistical Manual of Mental Disorders, Fifth Edition. Arlington, VA: American Psychiatric Association, 2013
2. King, V, Robinson S, Bianco T, et al. Choosing Antidepressants for Adults: Clinician's Guide. AHRQ Pub No. 07-EHC007-3 August 2007 www.effectivehealthcare.ahrq.gov
3. Acute and Longer-Term Outcomes in Depressed Outpatients Requiring One or Several Treatment Steps: A STAR*D Report: Am J Psychiatry 163:11, November 2006
4. Sequenced Treatment Alternatives to Relieve Depression (STAR*D): Lesson Learned: J Clin Psychiatry 69:7, July 2008
5. Effects of self poisoning with maprotiline. Knudsen K, Heath A Br Med J (Clin Res Ed). 1984 Feb;288(6417):601-3.
6. Skowron DM, Stimmel GL. Antidepressants and the risk of seizures. Pharmacotherapy 1992;12:18-22
7. Muzina, DJ. Discontinuing an antidepressant? Tapering tips to ease distressing symptoms. Current Psychiatry 2010 March; 9(3): 50-61
8. American Psychiatric Association. Practice guideline for the treatment of patients with major depressive disorder, 3rd ed. Arlington, Virginia: American Psychiatric Association, 2010
9. Cooper C, Katona C, Lyketsos K, Blazer D, Brodaty H, Rabins P, et al. A systematic review of treatments for refractory depression in older adults. Am J Psychiatry. 2011; 168; 681-8.
10. Gaynes BN, Dusetzina SB, Ellis AR, Hansen RA, Farley JF, Miller WC, et al. Treating depression after initial failure: directly comparing switch and augmenting strategies in STAR*D. J Clin Psychopharamcol. 2012; 32: 114-9.
11. Crome P, Braithwaite RA. Relationship between clinical features of tricyclic antidepressant poisoning and plasma concentrations in children. Arch Dis Child 1977;53:902–5.
12. Petit JM, Spiker DG, Ruwitch JF, Ruwich JF, Ziegler VE. Tricyclic antidepressant plasma levels and adverse effects after overdose. Clin Pharmacol Ther 1977;21:47–51.
13. Bailey DN, Van Dyke C, Langou RA, Jatlow PI. Tricyclic antidepressant; plasma levels and clinical findings in overdose. Am J Psychiatry 1978;135:1325–8.
14. Tricyclic Antidepressants ID and Quantitation http://www.questdiagnostics.com/testcenter/TestDetail.action?ntc=17482
15. Sheehan DV, Claycomb JB, Kouretas N. Monoamine oxidase inhibitors: prescription and patient management. *Int J Psychiatry Med*. 1980;10(2):99-121. [PubMed 7419369]
16. Mayo Clinic. (2013) Monamine oxidase inhibitors (MOAIs.) Retrieved January25, 2016 from http://www.mayoclinic.org/diseases-conditions/depression/expert-answers/maois/faq-20058035
17. American Psychiatric Association (APA). Treatment recommendations for patients with major depressive disorder. 3rd ed. May 2010. Available at http://psychiatryonline.org/pb/assets/raw/sitewide/practice_guidelines/guidelines/mdd.pdf
18. US Food and Drug Administration MedWatch Safety information. Available at: http://www.fda.gov/Drugs/DrugSafety/InformationbyDrugClass/UCM096273 Updated 12/23/14.

19. US Food and Drug Administration MedWatch Safety information. Available at: http://www.fda.gov/Safety/MedWatch/SafetyInformation/ucm409855.htm Updated 08/15/2014.

PACKAGE INSERTS:

TCA:

20. Sinequan® (doxepin) package insert. New York, NY. Pfizer; 2014 Jun.
21. Surmontil® (trimipramine maleate) package insert. East Hanover, NJ: Odyssey Pharmaceuticals, Inc.; 2001 Oct.
22. Amoxapine package insert. Corona, CA: Watson Laboratories, Inc.; 2014 Jun.
23. Pamelor (nortriptyline) package insert. Hazelwood, MO: Mallinckrodt, Inc.; 2014 May.
24. Surmontil (trimipramine maleate) package insert. East Hanover, NJ: Odyssey Pharmaceuticals, Inc.; 2014 Jul. 28759.
25. Ludiomil (maprotiline hydrochloride) package insert. Summit, NJ: Ciba-Geigy Corporation; 1996 Nov.
26. Tofranil-PM (imipramine pamoate) package insert. Hazelwood, MO: Mallinckrodt, Inc.; 2014 May.
27. Vivactil® (protriptyline) package insert. East Hanover, NJ: Odyssey Pharmaceuticals, Inc.; 2003 Jan.
28. Elavil® (amitriptyline) package insert. Wilmington, DE: AstraZeneca Pharmaceuticals LP; 2000 Dec.
29. Amitriptyline hydrochloride package insert. Princeton, NJ: Sandoz, Inc.; 2011 Jan.
30. Amitriptyline tablets package insert. Morgantown, WV: Mylan Pharmaceuticals, Inc.: 2014 Dec.
31. Anafranil® (clomipramine) package insert. St. Louis, MO; Mallinckrodt Inc.; 2001 Sep.

SSRI:

32. Celexa (citalopram) package insert. St. Louis, MO: Forest Pharmaceuticals, Inc.; 2014 Jul. 28270.
33. Lexapro (escitalopram) package insert. St. Louis, MO: Forest Pharmaceuticals, Inc.; 2014 Oct.
34. Luvox (fluvoxamine) package insert. Baudette, MN: ANI Pharmaceuticals, Inc.; 2014 Jul.
35. BRISDELLE® (paroxetine) package insert. Noven Therapeutics, LLC. Miami, FL 2014 Dec.
36. Paxil® (paroxetine HCL) package insert. Research Triangle Park, NC: GlaxoSmithKline; 2006 July.
37. Paxil CR (paroxetine hydrochloride) package insert. Research Triangle Park, NC: GlaxoSmithKline; 2014 Jul.
38. Pexeva (paroxetine mesylate) package insert. Miami, FL: Noven Therapeutics; 2014 Jul.
39. Paxil CR (paroxetine hydrochloride) package insert. Research Triangle Park, NC: GlaxoSmithKline; 2014 Jul.
40. Prozac (fluoxetine hydrochloride) package insert. Indianapolis, IN: Eli Lilly and Company; 2014 Oct.
41. Prozac (fluoxetine hydrochloride delayed release capsules) package insert. Indianapolis, IN: Eli Lilly and Company; 2014 Jul.
42. Sarafem (fluoxetine hydrochloride) package insert. Hunt Valley, MD: Pharmaceutics International, Inc. 2014 Oct.
43. Zoloft (sertraline) package insert. New York, NY: Pfizer; 2014 Aug.

SNRI:

44. Effexor® XR (venlafaxine extended-release) package insert. Philadelphia, PA; Wyeth Pharmaceuticals, Inc.; 2008 Jan.
45. Effexor® (venlafaxine) package insert. Philadelphia, PA; Wyeth Pharmaceuticals, Inc.; 2005 Dec.
46. Cymbalta (duloxetine hydrochloride) package insert. Indianapolis, IN: Eli Lilly and Company; 2015 Jun.
47. Irenka™ (duloxetine) package insert. Baltimore, MD: Lupin Pharma; 2015 May.
48. Pristiq (desvenlafaxine) extended-release tablets package insert. Philadelphia, PA: Wyeth Pharmaceuticals Inc.; 2014 Jul.
49. Khedezla™ (desvenlafaxine) package insert. Wilmington, NC. Osmotica Pharmaceutical Corp.: 2013 Jul.
50. Fetzima (levomilnacipran) extended-release capsules package insert. St. Louis, MO: Forest Laboratories, inc.; 2014 Jul.
51. Savella (milnacipran hydrochloride) tablets package insert. St Louis, MO: Forest Pharmaceuticals, Inc.; 2015 Jan.

DNRI:

52. Wellbutrin XL® (bupropion) package insert. Research Triangle Park, NC: GlaxoSmithKline; 2006 June
53. Wellbutrin SR (bupropion) package insert. Research Triangle Park, NC: GlaxoSmithKline; 2014 Jul.
54. Wellbutrin XL (bupropion) package insert. Bridgewater, NJ: BTA Pharmaceuticals, Inc.; 2014 Dec.
55. Wellbutrin (bupropion) package insert. Research Triangle Park, NC: GlaxoSmithKline; 2014 Jul.
56. Zyban (bupropion sustained release tablets) package insert. Research Triangle Park, NC: GlaxoSmithKline; 2014 Dec.
57. Aplenzin (bupropion extended release tablet) package insert. Bridgewater, NJ: Sanofi-aventis, LLC.; 2014 Jul.
58. Forfivo XL (bupropion hydrochloride extended-release tablets) package insert. Buffalo, NY: IntelGenx Corp; 2014 Jul.

5HT2 Antagonists:

59. Desyrel (trazodone) tablets. Morgantown, WV: Mylan Pharmaceuticals; 2014 Jul.
60. Oleptro (trazodone hydrochloride) extended-release tablets package insert. Dublin, Ireland: Labopharm Europe Limited; 2014 Jul.
61. Serzone® (nefazodone) package insert. Princeton, NJ: Bristol-Myers Squibb Company; 2003 Sep.

MAOI:

62. Marplan (isocarboxazid) package insert. Research Triangle Park, NC: GlaxoSmithKline; 2001 Aug.
63. Nardil (phenelzine) package insert. New York, NY: Pfizer; 2009 Feb.
64. Emsam (selegiline) transdermal system. Morgantown, WV: Somerset Pharmaceuticals, Inc.; 2015 Mar.
65. Parnate (tranylcypromine) package insert. Research Triangle Park, NC: GlaxoSmithKline; 2012 Jun.

Alpha 2 Antagonist:

66. Remeron (mirtazapine) package insert. Roseland, NJ: Organon USA, Inc.; 2015 Dec.
67. REMERON SolTab® (mirtazapine) package insert. Whitehouse Station, NJ: MERCK & Co., INC; 2014 Aug.

Miscellaneous antidepressants:

68. Viibryd (vilazodone) package insert. St. Louis, MO; Forest Pharmaceuticals, Inc.: 2015 Mar.
69. Trintellix (vortioxetine tablets) package insert. Deerfield, IL: Takeda Pharmacueticals America, Inc.; 2016 May.
70. US Food and Drug Administration MedWatch Safety information available at: http://www.fda.gov/Safety/MedWatch/SafetyInformation/SafetyAlertsforHumanMedicalProducts/ucm498607.htm Posted 05/02/2016.
71. Friedman RA. Antidepressants' black-box warning—10 years later. N Engl J Med. 2014; 371(18): 1666-8.
72. Funk, K, Bostwick, J. A Comparison of the Risk of QT Prolongation Among SSRIs. Annals of Pharmacotherapy47(10)1330–1341.
73. Desmarais, J, Looper, K. Interactions Between Tamoxifen and Antidepressants via Cytochrome P450 2D6. J Clin Psychiatry December 2009; 70:12 1688-1697.
74. Sideras, K, Ingle, J, Ames, M, et al. Coprescription of Tamoxifen and Medications That Inhibit CYP2D6: Recommendations Based on the Proposals by the Grading of Recommendations Assessment, Development, and Evaluation Working Group. J Clin Oncol. 2010; 1-9.
75. Cytochrome P450 drug interactions. Pharmacist's Letter/Prescriber's Letter 2006;22(2):220233.
76. Carlat, D. EMSAM: A User-Friendly MAOI? The Carlat Psychiatry Report. Vol 4 Number 11 Nov 2006. www.thecarlatreport.com
77. Comparison of Commonly Used Antidepressants. PHARMACIST'S LETTER / PRESCRIBER'S LETTER. 2008; 24 (3): 240509.
78. Comparison of venlafaxine and desvenlafaxine (Pristiq). Pharmacist's Letter/Prescriber's Letter 2009;25(2):250202.
79. Plattner, A Bezalel, D. The Tricyclics: More than Just Antidepressants. Psychiatric Annals 2011; 41(3): 158-165.
80. Ghose S, Haldar S. Therapeutic effort of doxepin in chronic idiopathic urticaria. Indian J Dermatol Venereol Leprol. 1990; 56(3): 218-220.
81. Montejo AL, Llorca G, Izquierdo JA, Rico-Villademoros F. Incidence of sexual dysfunction associated with antidepressant agents: a prospective multicenter study of 1022 outpatients. Spanish Working Group for the Study of Psychotropic-Related Sexual Dysfunction. J Clin Psychiatry. 2001;62 Suppl 3:10-21
82. Montejo-Gonzalez AL, Llorca G, Izquierdo JA, Ledesma A, et al. SSRI-induced sexual dysfunction: fluoxetine, paroxetine, sertraline, and fluvoxamine in a prospective, multicenter, and descriptive clinical study of 344 patients. J Sex Marital Ther. 1997 Fall;23(3):176-94
83. Handbook of Psychiatric Drug Therapy" Sixth Edition, by Labbate LA, et al. (Lippincott Williams & Wilkins, Philadelphia, 2010, 54-72)
84. Abilify (aripiprazole) tablets, discmelt orally-disintegrating tablets, oral solution, and intramuscular injection package insert. Princeton, NJ: Bristol-Myers Squibb Company; 2016 Aug.
85. Abilify Maintena (aripiprazole) extended-release intramuscular injection package insert. Rockville, MD:Otsuka America Pharmaceutical, Inc,; 2016 Aug.
86. Aristada (aripiprazole lauroxil) extended-release intramuscular suspension package insert. Waltham, MA: Alkermes, Inc.; 2016 Aug.
87. FDA Drug Safety Communication. FDA warns about new impulse-control problems associated with mental health drug aripiprazole (Abilify, Abilify Maintena, Aristada). Accessed on May 5, 2016. Available at: http://www.fda.gov/Drugs/DrugSafety/ucm498662.htm?source=govdelivery&utm_medium=email&utm_source=govdelivery.
88. Seroquel (quetiapine fumarate) package insert. Wilmington, DE: AstraZeneca Pharmaceuticals LP; 2016 Jun.
89. Seroquel XR (quetiapine fumarate extended-release tablets) package insert. Wilmington, DE: AstraZeneca Pharmaceuticals; 2016 Jun.
90. Symbyax (olanzapine; fluoxetine) package insert. Indianapolis, IN:Eli Lilly and Company; 2014 Oct.

Antipsychotics:

1. Antipsychotic Agents & Lithium. In: Trevor AJ, Katzung BG, Kruidering-Hall M. eds. *Katzung & Trevor's Pharmacology: Examination & Board Review, 11e* New York, NY: McGraw-Hill; 2015.
2. American Psychiatric Association. Diagnostic and Statistical Manual of Mental Disorder, Fifth Edition (DSM-5), American Psychiatric Association, Arlington, VA 2013.
3. Thorazine (chlorpromazine) Package Insert. Research Triangle Park, NC: GalaxoSmithKline; 2017 Mar.
4. Inapsine (droperidol) Package Insert. Lake Forest, IL: Akorn, Inc.; 2011 Nov.
5. Fluphenazine package insert. Princeton, NJ:Sandoz Inc.; 2017 Mar.
6. Fluphenazine decanoate injection package insert. Bedford, Ohio: Bedford Laboratories; 2017 Mar.
7. Fluphenazine hydrochloride solution for injection package insert. Schaumburg, Il:AAP Pharmaceuticals, LLC.; 2017 Mar. 17
8. Haldol Decanoate for Intramuscular Injection (haloperidol decanoate) package insert .Titusville, NJ: Janssen Pharmaceuticals, Inc,; 2017 Feb
9. Haloperidol tablets pacakge insert. Morgantown, WV: Mylan Pharmaceuticals Inc.; 2017 mar. 17.

10. Kreyenbuhl J, Buchanan RW, Dikerson FB, et al. The Schizophrenia Patient Outcomes Research Team (PORT): updataed treatment recommendations 2009. Schizophr Bull. 2010;36:94-103.

11. Moban (Molindone) package insert. Chadds Ford, PA: Endo Pharmaceuticals Inc; 2017 Mar.

12. Perphenazine package insert. Princeton, NJ: Sandoz Inc;2017 Mar.

13. Orap (pimozide) package insert. Sellersville, PA: Teva Pharmaceuticals USA; 2011 Nov.

14. Prochlorperazine suppositories package insert. South Plainfield, NJ: G&W Laboratories, Inc; 2016 Nov.

15. Prochlorperazine edisylate package insert. Eatonown, NJ: Heritage Pharmaceuticals Inc; 2013 Nov.

16. Mellaril (thioridazine) package insert. East Hanover, NJ: Novartis Pharmaceitucals Corporation; 2017 Mar.

17. Navane (thiothixene capsules) package insert. New York, NY : Pfizer, Inc .; 2017 Mar.

18. Trifluoperazine package insert. Princeton, NJ: Sanoz Inc; 2017 Mar.

19. Otani K, Aoshima T. Pharmacogenetics of classical and new antipsychotic drugs. *Ther Drug Monit* 2000;22:118-21.

20. Shin JG, Soukhova N, Flockhart DA. Effect of antipsychotic drugs on human liver cytochrome P-450 (CYP) isoforms in vitro: preferential inhibition of CYP2D6. *Drug Metab Dispos* 1999;27:1078-84.

21. Michalets EL. Update: clinically significant cytochrome P-450 drug interactions. *Pharmacotherapy* 1998;18:84-112.

22. Settle EC, Ayd FJ. Haloperidol: a quarter centry of experience. *J Clin Psychiatry* 1983;44:440-8.

23. Abilify (aripiprazole) tablets, discmelt orally-disintegrating tablets, oral solution, and intramuscular injection package insert. Princeton, NJ: Bristol-Myers Squibb Company; 2017 Mar.

24. Abilify Maintena (aripiprazole) extended-release intramuscular injection package insert. Rockville, MD:Otsuka America Pharmaceutical, Inc,;2017 Mar.

25. Aristada (aripiprazole lauroxil) extended-release intramuscular suspension package insert. Waltham, MA: Alkermes, Inc.;2016 Aug.

26. Saphris (asenapine) package isnert. St. Louis, MO: Forest Pharmaceuticals, Inc.; 2017 Mar.

27. Rexulti (brexpiprazole) tablets package insert. Rockville, MD: Otsuka Pharmaceutical Co., Ltd.; 2017 Mar.

28. Clozaril (clozapine) package insert. East Hanover, NJ: Novartis Pharmaceuticals, Corporation; 2017 Mar.

29. Fanapt (iloperidone) package insert. Rockville, MD: Vanda Pharmaceuticals, Inc.; 2017 Mar.

30. Latuda (lurasidone) package insert. Marlborough, MA: Sunovion Pharmaceuticals, Inc.; 2017 Mar.

31. Zyprexa (olanzapine, all formulations) package insert. Indianapolis, IN: Eli Lilly and Company; 2017 Mar.

32. Invega (paliperidone) package insert. Titusville, NJ: Janssen Pharmaceutica Products, L.P.; 2017 Mar.

33. Invega Sustenna (paliperidone palmitate injectable suspension) package insert. Titusville, NJ: Janssen Pharmaceuticals, Inc.; 2017 Mar.

34. Invega Trinza (paliperidone palmitate 3-month injectable suspension) package insert. Titusville, NJ: Janssen Pharmceuticals, Inc.; 2017 Mar.

35. Seroquel XR (quetiapine fumarate extended-release tablets) package insert. Wilmington, DE: AstraZeneca Pharmaceuticals; 2017 Mar.

36. Seroquel (quetiapine fumarate) package insert. Wilmington, DE: AstraZenca Pharmaceuticals LP; 2017 Mar.

37. Risperdal (risperidone tablets, oral solution, and orally disintegrating tablets) package insert. Titusville, NJ: Janssen Pharmaceuticals, Inc.; 2017 Feb.

38. Risperdal Consta (risperidone long-acting injection) package insert. Titusville, NJ: Janssen Pharmaceuticals, Inc.; 2017 Feb.

39. Geodon (ziprasidone) package insert. New York, NY: Pfizer: 2017 Mar.

40. Horacek J, Bubenikova-Valesova B, Kopecek M, et al. Mechanism of action of antipsychotic drugs and the neurobiology of schizophrenia. *CNS Drugs* 2006;20:389-409.

41. Llerena A, Berecz R, Penas-Lledo E. Pharmacogenetics of clinical response to risperidone. *Pharmacogenomics* 2013;14:177-194.

42. Nuplazid (pimavanserin) package insert. San Diego, CA: Acadia; 2016 Apr.

43. Chlorpromazine Hydrochloride Injection [prescribing information]. Eatontown, NJ: West-Ward Pharmaceuticals; November 2016.

44. McEvoy JP. Risks versus benefits of different types of long-acting injectable antipsychotics. *J Clin Psychiatry*. 2006;67(Suppl 5):15-18.

45. American Diabetes Association; American Psychiatric Association; American Association of Clinical Endocrinologists; North American Association for the Study of Obesity. Consensus development conference on antipsychotic drugs and obesity and diabetes. *J Clin Psychiatry*. 2004;65(2):267-272.

46. US Food and Drug Administration MedWatch Safety information. Available at: https://www.fda.gov/Drugs/DrugSafety/PostmarketDrugSafetyInformationforPatientsandProviders/ucm053171.htm

47. US Food and Drug Administration MedWatch Safety information. Available at: http://www.fda.gov/Drugs/DrugSafety/PostmarketDrugSafetyInformationforPatientsandProviders/ucm094303.htm. Updated 05/10/2016.

48. American Diabetes Association, American Psychiatric Association, American Association of Clinical Endocrinologists, North American Association for the Study of Obesity. Consensus development conference on antipsychotic drugs and obesity and diabetes. *Diabetes Care.* 2004; 27: 596-601.

49. Abilify® (aripiprazole) tablets, discmelt orally-disintegrating tablets, oral solution, and intramuscular injection. Rockville, MD: Otsuka America Pharmaceutical, Inc.; 2006 Sept.

50. Data on File. ABIMAI-007 (Unpublished data per Otsuka America Pharmaceutical, Inc.)

51. FDA Drug Safety Communication. FDA warns about new impulse-control problems associated with mental health drug aripiprazole (Abilify, Abilify Maintena, Aristada). Accessed on May 5, 2016. Available at: http://www.fda.gov.lp.hscl.ufl.edu/Drugs/DrugSafety/ucm498662.htm?source=govdelivery&utm_medium=email&utm_source=govdelivery.

52. Vraylar (cariprazine capsules) package insert. Parsippany, NJ:Actavis Pharma, Inc.; 2017 Mar.

53. FDA Drug Safety Communication: FDA modifies monitoring for neutropenia associated with schizophrenia medicine clozapine; approves new shared REMS program for all clozapine medicines. Accessed on September 15, 2015. Available on the world wide web at http://www.fda.gov/Drugs/DrugSafety/ucm461853.htm?source=govdelivery&utm_medium=email&utm_source=govdelivery.

54. Meltzer HY. Treatment of neuroleptic-nonresponsive schizophrenic patient. *Schizophr Bull.* 1992;18(3):515-542

55. Risperdal® (risperidone) package insert. Titusville, NJ: Janssen Pharmaceutica Products, L.P.; 2006 Oct.

56. Eerdekens M, Van Hove I, Remmerie B, et al. Pharmacokinetics and tolerability of long-acting risperidone in schizophrenia. *Schizophr Res* 2004;70:91-100.

57. J Psychiatr Pract. 2010 Mar;16(2):103-14. How sequential studies inform drug development: evaluating the effect of food intake on optimal bioavailability of ziprasidone. Lincoln J[1], Stewart ME, Preskorn SH.

58. CredibleMeds. QT drug lists. Available on the World Wide Web at http://www.crediblemeds.org.

59. Roden, DM. Drug-induced prolongation of the QT interval. *New Engl J Med* 2004;350:1013—22.

60. Zareba W, Lin DA. Antipsychotic drugs and QT interval prolongation. *Psychiatr Q* 2003;74:291—306.

61. Hansten PD, Horn JR. Drug Interactions with Drugs that Increase QTc Intervals. In: The Top 100 Drug Interactions - A Guide to Patient Management. 2007 Edition. Freeland, WA: H&H Publications; 2007:144-8.

62. Clozapine and the Risk of Neutropenia: An Overview for Healthcare Providers Available at: https://www.clozapinerems.com/CpmgClozapineUI/rems/pdf/resources/ANC_Table.pdf

63. Anderson RJ, Gambertoglio JG, & Schrier RWAnderson RJ, Gambertoglio JG, & Schrier RW: Clinical Use of Drugs in Renal Failure, Charles C Thomas, Springfield, IL, 1976.

64. Grunwald Z, Torjman M, Schieren H, et al: The pharmacokinetics of droperidol in anesthetized children.. Anesth Analg 1993; 76:1238-42.

65. Midha KK, Hawes EM, Hubbard JW, et al: Variation in the single dose pharmacokinetics of fluphenazine in psychiatric patients. Psychopharmacology (Berl) 1988; 96(2):206-211.

66. Simpson GM, Yadalam KG, Levinson DF, et al: Single-dose pharmacokinetics of fluphenazine after fluphenazine decanoate administration. J Clin Psychopharmacol 1990; 10:417-421.

67. Jann NW, Ereshefsky L, & Saklad SR: Clinical pharmacokinetics of the depot antipsychotics. Clin Pharmacokinetics 1985; 10:315-333.

68. Isah AO, Rawlins MD, & Bateman DN: Clinical pharmacology of prochlorperazine in healthy young males. Br J Clin Pharmacol 1991; 32:677-684.

69. Olver IN, Webster, LK, et al: A dose finding study of prochlorperazine as an antiemetic for cancer chemotherapy. Eur J Cancer Clin Oncol 1989; 25:1457-1461.

70. Taylor WB & Bateman DN: Preliminary studies of the pharmacokinetics and pharmacodynamics of prochlorperazine in healthy volunteers. Br J Clin Pharmacol 1987; 23:137-142.

71. Shvartsburd A, Sajadi C, Morton V, et al: Blood levels of haloperidol and thioridazine during maintenance neuroleptic treatment of schizophrenic outpatients. J Clin Psychopharmacol 1984a; 4:194-198.

72. Axelsson R: On the serum concentrations and antipsychotic effects of thioridazine, thioridazine side-chain sulfoxide and thioridazine side-chain sulfone, in chronic psychotic patients. Curr Ther Res 1977; 21:587.

73. Claghorn, JL. Review of clinical and laboratory experiences with molindone hydrochloride. J Clin Psychiatry 1985;46:30-3.

Bipolar Disorder, Antidpileptic Drugs & Mood Stabilizers:

1. American Psychiatric Association: Diagnostic and Statistical Manual of Mental Disorders, Fifth Edition. Arlington, VA: American Psychiatric Association, 2013

2. *2015 Florida Best Practice Psychotherapeutic Medication Guidelines for Adults* (2015). The University of South Florida, Florida Medicaid Drug Therapy Management Program sponsored by the Florida Agency for Health Care

Administration. Available at: http://www.medicaidmentalhealth.org/_assets/file/Guidelines/Web_2015-Psychotherapeutic%20Medication%20Guidelines%20for%20Adults_Final_Approved1.pdf

3. Yatham LN, Kennedy SH, Schaffer A, Parikh SV, Beaulieu S, O_Donovan C, MacQueen G, McIntyre RS, Sharma V, Ravindran A, Young LT, Young AH, Alda M, Milev R, Vieta E, Calabrese JR, Berk M, Ha K, Kapczinski F. Canadian Network for Mood and Anxiety Treatments (CANMAT) and International Society for Bipolar Disorders (ISBD) collaborative update of CANMAT guidelines for the management of patients with bipolar disorder: update 2009. Bipolar Disord 2009: 11: 225–255. Available at: http://www.canmat.org/resources/canmat%20bipolar%20disorder%20guidelines%20-2009%20update.pdf

4. American Psychiatric Association (2002). Practice guideline for the treatment of patients with bipolar disorder (revision). American Journal of Psychiatry, 159(4, Suppl):1-82. Available at: https://psychiatryonline.org/pb/assets/raw/sitewide/practice_guidelines/guidelines/bipolar.pdf

5. Suppes T, Dennehy E, Hirschfeld RMA, Altshuler LL, Bowden CL, Calíbrese CR, Crismon ML, Ketter T, Sachs G, Swann AC. The Texas Implementation of Medication Algorithms: Update to the Algorithms for Treatment of Bipolar I Disorder. *J Clin Psychiatr*y 2005; 60:870-886. Available at: https://www.jpshealthnet.org/sites/default/files/tmap_bipolar_2007.pdf

6. US Food and Drug Administration MedWatch Safety information. Available at: http://www.fda.gov/Drugs/DrugSafety/PostmarketDrugSafetyInformationforPatientsandProviders/ucm094303.htm. Updated 05/10/2016.

7. US Food and Drug Administration MedWatch Safety information. Available at: http://www.fda.gov/Drugs/DrugSafety/PostmarketDrugSafetyInformationforPatientsandProviders/ucm100190.htm. Updated 05/05/2009.

8. American Diabetes Association, American Psychiatric Association, American Association of Clinical Endocrinologists, North American Association for the Study of Obesity. Consensus development conference on antipsychotic drugs and obesity and diabetes. *Diabetes Care.* 2004; 27: 596-601.

9. Abilify (aripiprazole) tablets, discmelt orally-disintegrating tablets, oral solution, and intramuscular injection package insert. Princeton, NJ: Bristol-Myers Squibb Company; 2016 Aug.

10. Abilify Maintena (aripiprazole) extended-release intramuscular injection package insert. Rockville, MD:Otsuka America Pharmaceutical, Inc,; 2016 Aug.

11. Aristada (aripiprazole lauroxil) extended-release intramuscular suspension package insert. Waltham, MA: Alkermes, Inc.; 2016 Aug.

12. FDA Drug Safety Communication. FDA warns about new impulse-control problems associated with mental health drug aripiprazole (Abilify, Abilify Maintena, Aristada). Accessed on May 5, 2016. Available at: http://www.fda.gov/Drugs/DrugSafety/ucm498662.htm?source=govdelivery&utm_medium=email&utm_source=govdelivery.

13. Food and Drug Administration Medwatch. Antipsychotic drugs: Class labeling change - Treatment during pregnancy and potential risk to newborns. Retrieved February 22, 2001. Available on the World Wide Web http://www.fda.gov/Safety/MedWatch/SafetyInformation/SafetyAlertsforHumanMedicalProducts/ucm244175.htm.

14. Winans E. Aripiprazole. *Am J Health Syst Pharm.* 2003;60:2437—45.

15. Casey DE, Carson WH, Saha AR, et al. on behalf of the Aripiprazole Study Group. Switching patients to aripiprazole from other antipsychotic agents: a multicenter randomized study. Psychopharmacology 2003;166:391-9.

16. Hadjakis WJ, Marcus R, Abou-Gharbia N, et al. Aripiprazole in acute mania: results from a second placebo-controlled study. Bipolar Disord 2004;6 Suppl 1:39-40.

17. Saphris (asenapine) package insert. St. Loius, MO: Forest Pharmaceuticals, Inc.; 2015 Mar. 60164.

18. Vraylar (cariprazine capsules) package insert. Parsippany, NJ:Actavis Pharma, Inc.;2015 Sept.

19. Carbatrol (carbamazepine extended release capsules) package insert. Lexington, MA: Shire US Inc.; 2015 Nov.

20. Tegretol (carbamazepine) package insert. East Hanover, NJ: Novartis Pharmaceuticals Corporation; 2015 Sep.

21. CARNEXIV [package insert]. Deerfield, IL: Lundbeck. **2.** Tolbert D, Cloyd J, Biton V, et al. Bioequivalence of oral and intravenous carbamazepine formulations in adult patients with epilepsy. *Epilepsia.* 2015:56(6):915-923.

22. Chlorpromazine package insert. Princeton, NJ: Sandoz Inc; 2010 Sept.

23. Depakote® (Divalproex Sodium Delayed-Release tablets) package insert. North Chicago, IL: Abbott Laboratories; 2003 Sept.

24. Depakote® ER (Divalproex Sodium Extended-Release tablets) package insert. North Chicago, IL: Abbott Laboratories; 2006 April.

25. Depakene (valproic acid) prescribing information. North Chicago, IL: Abbott Laboratories; 2009 April.

26. Equetro (carbamazepine extended release capsules) package insert. Parsippany, NJ: Validus Pharmaceuticals LLC; 2012 Nov.

27. Neurontin (gabapentin) package insert. New York, NY: Parke Davis; 2015 Sep.

28. Pande AC, Crockatt JG, Janney CA, et al. Gabapentin in bipolar disorder: a placebo-controlled trial of adjunctive therapy. Gabapentin Bipolar Disorder Study Group. Bipolar Disord 2000;2(3 Pt 2):249-55.

29. Eur Psychiatry. 2000 Nov;15(7):433-7.Adjunctive gabapentin treatment of bipolar disorder.

30. L.T Young, J.C Robb, I Patelis-Siotis, C MacDonald, R.T Joffe. Acute treatment of bipolar depression with gabapentin. Biol Psychiatry, 42 (1997), pp. 851–853

31. Gralise (gabapentin) extended-release tablets. Menlo Park, CA: Depomed Inc; 2012 Apr.

32. Horizant (gabapentin enacarbil) extended-release tablets. Research Triangle Park, NC: GlaxoSmithKline; 2013 May.

33. Trileptal (oxcarbazepine) package insert. East Hanover, NJ: Novartis Pharmaceuticals Corporation; 2014 Jul.
34. Oxtellar XR (oxcarbazepine) extended-release tablets. Rockville, MD: Supernus Pharmaceuticals; 12 Oct.
35. Wagner KD, Kowatch RA, Emslie GJ, et al. A double-blind, randomized, placebo-controlled trial of oxcarbazepine in the treatment of bipolar disorder in children and adolescents. Am J Psychiatry. 2006;163:1179-1186. Erratum in: Am J Psychiatry 2006;163:1843.
36. Vasudev A, Macritchie K, Vasudev K, et al. Oxcarbazepine for acute affective episodes in bipolar disorder. Cochrane Database Syst Rev. 2011 Dec 7;(12):CD004857. doi: 10.1002/14651858.CD004857.pub2.
37. Kakkar AK, Rehan HS, Unni KE, et al. Comparative efficacy and safety of oxcarbazepine versus divalproex sodium in the treatment of acute mania: a pilot study. Eur Psychiatry 2009;24:178-82.
38. Crismon ML, Argo TR, Bendele SD, et al. Texas Medication Algorithm Project procedural manual. Bipolar Disorder Algorithms. Texas Department of State Health Services 2007.
39. Loxapine package insert. Morgantown, WV: Mylan Pharmaceuticals Inc.; 2010 Sept.
40. Adasuve (loxapine inhalation powder) package insert. Mountain View, CA: Alexza Pharmaceuticals, Inc.; 2012 Dec.
41. Risperdal® (risperidone) package insert. Titusville, NJ: Janssen Pharmaceutica Products, L.P.; 2006 Oct.
42. Trileptal (oxcarbazepine) package insert. East Hanover, NJ: Novartis Pharmaceuticals Corporation; 2014 Jul.
43. Geodon® (ziprasidone) package insert. New York, NY: Pfizer: 2015 Aug.
44. J Clin Psychiatry. 2009 Jan;70(1):58-62. Epub 2008 Oct 21.
    The impact of calories and fat content of meals on oral ziprasidone absorption: a randomized, open-label, crossover trial.
45. Lamictal (lamotrigine) package insert. Research Triangle Park, NC: GlaxoSmithKline; 2015 May.
46. Lamictal XR (lamotrigine extended-release tablet) package insert. Research Triangle Park, NC: GlaxoSmithKline; 2015 Mar.
47. Food and Drug Administration (US FDA) MedWatch. Lamictal (lamotrigine): label change - risk of aseptic meningitis. Retrieved August 13, 2010. Available on the World Wide Web at http://www.fda.gov/Safety/MedWatch/SafetyInformation/SafetyAlertsforHumanMedicalProducts/ucm222269.htm.
48. Lithium carbonate tablets, lithium carbonate capsules USP, lithium oral solution USP package insert. Columbus, Ohio; Roxane: 2011 Sept.
49. Lithobid extended-release tablets (lithium carbonate, USP) package insert. Miami, FL: Noven Therapeutics, LLC; 2016 Jun.
50. American Journal of Pharmaceutical Education 2005; 69 (5) Article 88.
51. Finley PR. Drug interactions with lithium: an update. Clin Pharmacokinet 2016; 55:925-41.
52. Eskalith (lithium carbonate) package insert. Research Triangle Park, NC: GlaxoSmithKline; 2003 Sept.
53. Zyprexa (olanzapine, all formulations) package insert. Indianapolis, IN: Eli Lilly and Company; 2015 Jul.
54. Symbyax (olanzapine; fluoxetine) package insert. Indianapolis, IN:Eli Lilly and Company; 2014 Oct.
55. Zyprexa Relprevv (olanzapine for extended-release injectable suspension) package insert. Indianapolis, IN: Eli Lilly and Company; 2015 Jul
56. US Food and Drug Administration (FDA). FDA Safety Communication: FDA warns about rare but serious skin reactions with mental health drug olanzapine (Zyprexa, Zyprexa Zydis, Zyprexa Relprevv, and Symbyax). May 2016. Retrieved May 10, 2016. Available on the World Wide Web at: http://www.fda.gov/Drugs/DrugSafety/ucm499441.htm?source=govdelivery&utm_medium=email&utm_source=govdelivery
57. Tohen, Vieta E, Calabrese J, et al. Efficacy of olanzapine and olanzapine-fluoxetine combination in the treatment of bipolar I depression. Arch Gen Psychiatry 2003;60:1079-88.
58. Berk M, Dodd S. Efficacy of atypical antipsychotics in bipolar disorder. Drugs 2005;65:257-69.
59. Fanapt (iloperidone) package insert. Rockville, MD: Vanda Pharmaceuticals, Inc.; 2016 May.
60. Latuda (lurasidone) package insert. Fort Lee, NJ: Sunovion Pharmaceuticals, Inc.; 2013 Jul.
61. Chlorpromazine package insert. Princeton, NJ: Sandoz Inc; 2010 Sept.
62. Topamax (topiramate) package insert. Titusville, NJ: Janssen Pharmaceuticals, Inc.; 2014 Dec.
63. Topamax® (topiramate) package insert. Raritan, NJ: Ortho-McNeil Pharmaceutical, Inc.; 2005 June.
64. Qudexy XR (topiramate) package insert. Maple Grove, MN: Upsher-Smith Laboratories; 2015 Mar.
65. Trokendi XR (topiramate extended-release capsules) package insert. Rockville, MD: Supernus Pharmaceuticals; 2016 Aug.
66. Risperdal (risperidone) package insert. Titusville, NJ: Janssen Pharmaceuticals, Inc.; 2016 Mar.
67. Risperdal Consta (risperidone long-acting injection) package insert. Titusville, NJ: Janssen Pharmaceuticals, Inc.; 2016 Mar.
68. Approved Risk Evaluation and Mitigation Strategies (REMS) via REMS@FDA Available at: http://www.accessdata.fda.gov/scripts/cder/rems/index.cfm
69. Seroquel (quetiapine fumarate) package insert. Wilmington, DE: AstraZeneca Pharmaceuticals LP; 2016 Jun.
70. Seroquel XR (quetiapine fumarate extended-release tablets) package insert. Wilmington, DE: AstraZeneca Pharmaceuticals; 2016 Jun.

Attention Deficit Hyperactivity Disorder, Narcolepsy/Somnolence

1. American Psychiatric Association: Diagnostic and Statistical Manual of Mental Disorders, Fifth Edition. Arlington, VA: American Psychiatric Association, 2013

2. Mayo Clinic. (2013) Adult ADHD (attention-deficit/hyperactivity disorder.) Retrieved February 20, 2016 from http://www.mayoclinic.org/diseases-conditions/adult-adhd/basics/definition/con-20034552

3. American Psychiatric Association (APA). Treatment recommendations for patients with major depressive disorder. 3rd ed. May 2010. Available at http://psychiatryonline.org/pb/assets/raw/sitewide/practice_guidelines/guidelines/mdd.pdf

4. US Food and Drug Administration MedWatch Safety information. Available at: http://www.fda.gov/drugs/drugsafety/postmarketdrugsafetyinformationforpatientsandproviders/drugsafetyinformationforheathcareprofessionals/ucm165858.htm Updated 08/15/2013.

5. US Food and Drug Administration MedWatch Safety information. Available at: http://www.fda.gov/safety/medwatch/safetyinformation/ucm381078.htm. Updated 1/10/2014.

6. Food and Drug Administration Drug Safety Communication. Safety review update of medications used to treat attention-deficit/hyperactivity disorder (ADHD) in children and young adults. Retrieved April 01, 2016. Available on the World Wide Web http://www.fda.gov/Drugs/DrugSafety/ucm277770.htm#data.

7. Institute for Safe Medication Practices (ISMP). ISMP Medication Safety Alert: Adverse drug events in children less than 18 years old. Retrieved from the World Wide Web February 25, 2014. Available at: http://www.ismp.org/Newsletters/acutecare/showarticle.aspx?id=67

8. Davis JM, Kopin IJ, Lemberger L, et al. Effects of urinary pH on amphetamine metabolism. Ann N Y Acad Sci 1971;179:493-501.

9. Linden CH, Kulig KW, Rumack BH. Amphetamines. Top Emerg Med 1985;7:18-32.

10. Baselt RC, Cravey RH. Amphetamine. In: Disposition of Toxic Drugs and Chemicals in Man. Foster City, CA: Chemical Toxicology Institute 1995;44-47.

11. Adderall® (amphetamine; dextroamphetamine) package insert. Newport, KY: Shire US Inc.; 2005 March.

12. Adderall XR® (amphetamine; dextroamphetamine) package insert. Wayne, PA: Shire US Inc.; 2015 Apr.

13. Adderall® (amphetamine; dextroamphetamine) package insert. Horsham, PA: Teva Select Brands; 2015 Oct.

14. Adzenys (amphetamine) XR-ODT tablet package insert. Grand Prairie, TX: Neos Therapeutics LP; 2016 Jan.

15. Cassels, Caroline. FDA Okays First Orally Disintegrating Tablet for ADHD in Kids. Medscape 2016. Retrieved January 28, 2016. Available at: http://www.medscape.com/viewarticle/857892?nlid=98264_3901&src=wnl_newsalrt_160128_MSCPEDIT&uac=174991HV&impID=972066&faf=1

16. DYANAVEL XR (amphetamine) extended-release oral suspension package insert, Tris Pharma, Inc.; 2015 Nov.

17. Dexedrine® (dextroamphetamine) package insert. Research Triangle Park, NC; GlaxoSmithKline; 2007 Mar.

18. Dexedrine Spansule® (dextroamphetamine sustained-release capsules) package insert. Winchester, KY: Catalent Pharma Solutions; 2015 Apr.

19. Desoxyn® (methamphetamine hydrochloride) package insert. Deerfield, IL: Ovation Pharmaceuticals, Inc.; 2007 May.

20. Vyvanse (lisdexamfetamine) package insert. Wayne, PA: Shire US Inc.; 2015 Apr.

21. Zenzedi (dextroamphetamine sulfate) tablet package insert. Atlanta, GA: Arbor Pharmaceuticals, LLC; 2013 May.

22. Aptensio XR (methylphenidate hydrochloride) capsule package insert. Greenville, NC: Pantheon: 2015 Apr.

23. Concerta (methylphenidate hydrochloride) package insert. Vacaville, CA: Janssen Pharmaceuticals, Inc.; 2015 Apr.

24. Daytrana™ (methylphenidate transdermal system) package insert. Wayne, PA: Shire Pharmaceuticals US Inc.; 2006 Apr

25. Daytrana (methylphenidate transdermal system) package insert. Miami, FL: Noven Therapeutics, LLC; 2015 Aug.

26. FDA Drug Safety Communication. FDA reporting permanent skin color changes associated with use of Daytrana patch (methylphenidate transdermal system) for treating ADHD. Retrieved June 24, 2015. Available on the World Wide Web at http://www.fda.gov/Drugs/DrugSafety/ucm452244.htm?source=govdelivery&utm_medium=email&utm_source=govdelivery.

27. Focalin® (dexmethylphenidate) package insert. East Hanover, NJ: Novartis Pharmaceutical Corp.; 2007 Apr

28. Metadate CD™ (methylphenidate extended-release) package insert. Smyrna, GA: UCB, Inc.; 2015 Feb.

29. Metadate ER (methylphenidate extended release) package insert. Smyrna, GA; UCB, Inc. 2014 Aug.

30. Methylin (methylphenidate chewable tablet) package insert. Hazelwood, MO: Mallinckrodt Inc.; 2015 Feb.
31. Methylin (methylphenidate oral solution) package insert. Hazelwood, MO: Mallinckrodt Inc.; 2015 Feb.
32. Quillivant XR (methylphenidate hydrochloride) extended-release oral suspension. New York, NY: Pfizer Inc.; 2015 Feb.
33. QuilliChew ER (methylphenidate) chewable tablets package insert. Monmouth Junction, NJ: Tris Pharma, Inc.; 2015 Dec.
34. Ritalin LA® (methylphenidate) package insert. East Hanover, NJ: Novartis Pharmaceutical Corp.; 2004 Apr.
35. Ritalin LA® (methylphenidate) package insert. East Hanover, NJ: Novartis Pharmaceutical Corp.; 2015 Apr., Inc.; 2015 Apr.
36. Ritalin® and Ritalin SR® (methylphenidate) package insert. East Hanover, NJ: Novartis Pharmaceutical Corp.; 2015 Apr.
37. Wellbutrin XL® (bupropion) package insert. Research Triangle Park, NC: GlaxoSmithKline; 2006 June
38. Wellbutrin SR (bupropion) package insert. Research Triangle Park, NC: GlaxoSmithKline; 2014 Jul.
39. Wellbutrin XL (bupropion) package insert. Bridgewater, NJ: BTA Pharmaceuticals, Inc.; 2014 Dec.
40. Wellbutrin (bupropion) package insert. Research Triangle Park, NC: GlaxoSmithKline; 2014 Jul.
41. Zyban (bupropion sustained release tablets) package insert. Research Triangle Park, NC: GlaxoSmithKline; 2014 Dec.
42. Aplenzin (bupropion extended release tablet) package insert. Bridgewater, NJ: Sanofi-aventis, LLC.; 2014 Jul.
43. Forfivo XL (bupropion hydrochloride extended-release tablets) package insert. Buffalo, NY: IntelGenx Corp; 2014 Jul.
44. Strattera (atomoxetine) package insert. Indianapolis, IN: Eli Lilly and Company;2015 Apr.
45. Xyrem (sodium oxybate) oral solution package insert. Minnetonka, MN: Orphan Medical, Inc.; 2015 Apr.
46. Evekeo (amphetamine sulfate tablets) package insert. Atlanta, GA: Arbor Pharmaceuticals, LLC: 2015 Apr.
47. Nuvigil™ (armodafinil) package insert. Frazer, PA: Cephalon, Inc; 2013 Jun.
48. Provigil® (modafinil) package insert. West Chester, PA: Cephalon, Inc; 2004 Feb.
49. Catapres® tablets (clonidine) package insert. Ridgefield, CT: Boehringer Ingelheim Pharmaceuticals, Inc.; 2016 Aug.
50. Catapres (clonidine) extended-release patch. Ridgefield, CT: Boehringer Ingelheim Pharmaceuticals, Inc.; 2016 Aug.
51. Kapvay (clonidine hydrochloride) extended-release tablets package insert. St. Michael, Barbados: Concordia Pharmaceuticals Inc.; 2016 Aug.
52. Intuniv (guanfacine) package insert. Lexington, MA: Shire US Inc.; 2016 Mar.
53. Guanfacine hydrochloride tablet package insert. Morgantown, WV: Mylan Pharmaceuticals Inc.; 2003 Apr.
54. Tenex (guanfacine) package insert. Bridgewater, NJ: Promius Pharma, LLC; 2013 July.
55. Markowitz JS, Patrick KS. Pharmacokinetic and pharmacodynamic drug interactions in the treatment of attention-deficit hyperactivity disorder. Clin Pharmacokinet 2001;40:753-72.
56. Handbook of Psychiatric Drug Therapy" Sixth Edition, by Labbate LA, et al. (Lippincott Williams & Wilkins, Philadelphia, 2010, 265-282)
57. Institute for Clinical Systems Improvement. Attention Deficit Hyperactivity Disorder in Primary Care for School Age Children and Adolescents, Diagnosis and Management of. Retrieved November 08, 2016. Available at https://www.icsi.org/_asset/60nzr5/ADHD-Interactive0312.pdf
58. MTA Cooperative Group. National Institute of Mental Health Multimodal Treatment Study of ADHD follow-up: changes in effectiveness and growth after the end of treatment. Pediatrics 2004;113:762—9
59. Davis JM, Kopin IJ, Lemberger L, et al. Effects of urinary pH on amphetamine metabolism. Ann N Y Acad Sci 1971;179:493—501.
60. American Academy of Pediatrics subcommittee on attention-deficit/hyperactivity disorder, steering committee on quality improvement and management. ADHD: clinical practice guideline for the diagnosis, evaluation, and treatment of attention-deficit/hyperactivity disorder in children and adolescents. Pediatrics 2011;128(5):1007-1022.
61. Dopheide JQ, Pliszka SR. Attention-deficit-hyperactivity disorder: an update. Pharmacotherapy 2009;29:656-679.

Substance Abuse

1. American Psychiatric Association: Diagnostic and Statistical Manual of Mental Disorders, Fifth Edition. Arlington, VA: American Psychiatric Association, 2013
2. Gourlay DL, Heit HA, Caplan YH. Urine Drug Testing in Clinical Practice: The Art and Science of Patient Care. Johns Hopkins Medicine. 2012; 5: Available at: http://eo2.commpartners.com/users/ama/downloads/udt5_Copy.pdf Accessed on: 2014-01-02.
3. ReVia (naltrexone hydrochloride) package insert. Pomona, NY: Duramed Pharmaceuticals, Inc. 2013 Oct.
4. Vivitrol (naltrexone extended release injectable suspension) package insert. Cambridge, MA: Alkermes, Inc.; 2015 Dec.
5. Naltrexone (naltrexone hydrochloride) package insert. Hazelwood, MO: Mallinckrodt, Inc. 2009 Feb.

6. Antabuse (disulfiram) tablet package insert. Pomona, NY: Duramed Pharmaceuticals, Inc.; 2010 Feb.

7. Campral (acamprosate calcium) package insert. St. Louis, MO: Forest Pharmaceuticals, Inc.; 2012 Jan.

8. Dolophine (methadone) package insert. Columbus, OH: Roxane Laboratories, Inc; 2015 Apr.

9. Methadose Oral Concentrate and Methadose Sugar-Free Oral Concentrate (methadone hydrochloride oral concentrate USP) package insert. Hazelwood, MO: Mallinckrodt Inc.; 2009 Oct.

10. Methadone tablets for oral suspension (methadone Diskets). Columbus, OH: Boehringer Ingelheim Roxane Laboratories; 2013 Sept.

11. Methadone oral solution package insert. Columbus, OH: Roxane Laboratories: 2014 Apr.

12. Methadone Hydrochloride Injection package insert. Wilmington, NC: AAI Pharma; 2004 Feb.

13. Buprenorphine; naloxone sublingual tablets package insert. North Wales, PA: Teva Pharmaceuticals, USA; 2014 Dec.

14. Suboxone® (buprenorphine and naloxone)/Subutex® (buprenorphine) package insert. Richmond, VA: Reckitt Benckiser Pharmaceuticals, Inc.; 2006 Sep.

15. Suboxone (buprenorphine and naloxone) sublingual tablets package insert. Richmond, VA: Reckitt Benckiser Pharmaceuticals, Inc.; 2011 Dec.

16. Suboxone (buprenorphine; naloxone) sublingual film package insert. Richmond, VA: Reckitt Benckiser Pharmaceuticals, Inc.; 2015 Sept.

17. Suboxone® (buprenorphine and naloxone)/Subutex® (buprenorphine) package insert. Richmond, VA: Reckitt Benckiser Pharmaceuticals, Inc.; 2006 Sep.

18. Zubsolv (buprenorphine; naloxone) sublingual tablets package insert. Chadds Ford, PA: Orexo AB; 2015 Aug.

19. Bunavail (buprenorphine; naloxone) buccal film package insert. Raleigh, NC: BioDelivery Sciences International, Inc.; 2014 June.

20. Belbuca (buprenorphine) buccal film package insert. Endo Pharmaceuticals Inc.: Malvern, PA; 2015 Oct.

21. Buprenex® (buprenorphine) package insert. Richmond, VA: Reckitt Benckiser Pharmaceuticals, Inc.; 2001 Jul.

22. Buprenorphine sublingual tablets package insert. Elizabeth, NJ: Actavis Elizabeth, LLC.; 2015 Jan

23. Butrans (buprenorphine transdermal system) package insert. Stamford, CT: Purdue Pharma L.P.; 2014 Jun.

24. Buprenex (buprenorphine hydrochloride) injection, solution package insert. Richmond, VA: Reckitt Benckiser Pharmaceuticals, Inc.; 2014 Feb.

25. Probuphine (buprenorphine) implant package insert. Princeton, NJ: Braeburn Pharmaceuticals, Inc.; 2016 May.

26. National Institutes of Health (NIH). Buprenorphine monograph. LactMed: Drug and Lactation Database. Available at http://toxnet.nlm.nih.gov.lp.hscl.ufl.edu/cgi-bin/sis/search2/f?./temp/~1F4u8f:1. Accessed November 16, 2015.

27. Buprenorphine. Substance Abuse and Mental Health Services Administration (SAMHSA). Retrieved from the World Wide Web August 4, 2016 at http://www.samhsa.gov/medication-assisted-treatment/treatment/buprenorphine.

28. Food and Drug Administration (FDA). FDA Drug Safety Communication: FDA warns about serious risks and death when combining opioid pain or cough medicines with benzodiazepines; requires its strongest warning. http://www.fda.gov/Drugs/DrugSafety/ucm518473.htm. Retrieved August 31, 2016

29. Evzio (naloxone hydrochloride injection) package insert. Richmond, VA: Kaleo, Inc.; 2016 Oct Narcan

30. Narcan (naloxone hydrochloride) nasal spray package insert. Radner, PA: Adapt Pharma, Inc.;2015 Nov. Narcan (naloxone hydrochloride injection, USP) package insert. Chadds Ford, PA: Endo Pharmaceuticals Inc.; 2003 Jul.

31. Naloxone package insert. Lake Forest, IL: Hospira Inc.; 2008 Jan.

32. National Practice Guideline for the Use of Medications in the Treatment of Addiction Involving Opioid Use. Available at: http://www.asam.org/docs/default-source/practicesupport/guidelines-and-consensus-docs/national-practice-guideline.pdf. Accessed: June 4, 2015

33. Management of Substance Use Disorders Work Group. VA/DoD clinical practice guideline for the management of substance use disorders. Version 3.0. Washington (DC): Department of Veterans Affairs, Department of Defense; 2015 Dec. 169 p. [327 references] Available at: http://www.healthquality.va.gov/guidelines/MH/sud/VADoDSUDCPGRevised22216.pdf

34. Prostep (nicotine) package insert. Advantus Pharm & Lederle Lab Div. Peral River, NY. 1992.

35. Commit (nicotine) package insert. GlaxoSmithKline Healthcare. Pittsburgh, PA

36. Nicotrol NS (nicotine nasal spray) package insert. New York, NY: Pharmacia and Upjohn Company; 2013 Jun.

37. Nicotrol Inhaler (nicotine inhalation system) package insert. New York, NY: Pharmacia & Upjohn Co; 2008 Dec.

38. Nicorette (nicotine polacrilex gum) consumer labeling. Moon Townshipe, PA; GlaxoSmithKline Consumer Healthcare, LP: 2014 Jun.

39. Stead LF, Perera R, Bullen C, et al. Nicotine replacement therapy for smoking cessation. Cochrane Database Syst Rev 2012 Nov 14;11:CD000146. doi: 10.1002/14651858.CD000146.pub4.Review.

40. Nicorette (nicotine polacrilex lozenge) consumer labeling. Moon Township, PA; GlaxoSmithKline Consumer Healthcare, L.P.: 2015 May.

41. Nicoderm CQ (nicotine) transdermal patch consumer labeling. Moon Township, PA; GlaxoSmithKline Consumer Healthcare, L.P.: 2015 Oct.

42. Habitrol (nicotine transdermal patch) consumer labeling. Parsippany, NJ: Novartis Consumer Health; 2014 July.

43. U.S. Food and Drug Administration (FDA). FDA Consumer Updates: Nicotine replacement therapy labels may change. Published April 1, 2013. Available at: www.fda.gov/ForConsumers/ConsumerUpdates/ucm345087.htm#2 Accessed: Jan 7, 2014.

44. Institute for Safe Medication Practices (ISMP). Burns during MRI from patches with metal in the backing. Acute Care ISMP Medication Safety Alert 2016;21:1-2.

45. Chantix (varenicline) package insert. New York, NY: Pfizer Labs; 2016 Dec.
46. Zyban (bupropion sustained release tablets) package insert. Research Triangle Park, NC: GlaxoSmithKline; 2016 Jun.
47. Gowing L, Farrell MF, Ali R, et al. Alpha2-adrenergic agonists for the management of opioid withdrawal. Cochrane Database Syst Rev. 2014 Mar 31;3:CD002024. doi:10.1002/14651858.CD002024.pub4.

Weight Loss & Miscellaneous
1. Bachorik L. FDA announces withdrawal of fenfluramine and dexfenfluramine. HHS News. P97-32. Food and Drug Administration; 1997 Sep 15
2. N Engl J Med 1997 Aug 28; 337(9): 581-8. Valvular heart disease associated with fenfluramine-phentermine.
3. U.S. Food and Drug Administration. FDA ISSUES PUBLIC HEALTH WARNING ON PHENYLPROPANOLAMINE. Last update 12/07/2015. Available at http://www.fda.gov/Drugs/DrugSafety/InformationbyDrugClass/ucm150763.htm
4. Meridia® (sibutramine) package insert. North Chicago, IL: Abbott Laboratories; 2003 Oct.
5. FDA Drug Safety Communication: FDA Recommends Against the Continued Use of Meridia (sibutramine.) Last update 3/25/2016. Available at http://www.fda.gov/Drugs/DrugSafety/ucm228746.htm
6. Evekeo (amphetamine sulfate tablets) package insert. Atlanta, GA: Arbor Pharmaceuticals, LLC: 2015 Apr.
7. Didrex® (benzphetamine) package insert. Kalamazoo, MI; Pharmacia and Upjohn Company; 2002 Apr.
8. Regimex™ (benzphetamine) package insert. Ridgeland, MS; WraSer Pharmaceuticals; 2012 Sept.
9. Tenuate® (diethylpropion hydrochloride) package insert. Bridgewater, NJ: Aventis Pharmaceuticals; 2003 Nov.
10. Phendimetrazine tartrate extended-release capsules package insert. Laurelton, NY: Eon Labs Manufacturing, Inc.; 1994 Apr.
11. Phendimetrazine tartrate extended-release capsules package insert. Princeton, NJ: Sandoz Inc.; 2011 Oct.
12. Desoxyn® (methamphetamine hydrochloride) package insert. Deerfield, IL: Ovation Pharmaceuticals, Inc.; 2007 May.
13. Desoxyn (methamphetamine hydrochloride) package insert. Deerfield, IL: Abbott Pharmaceuticals, Inc.; 2013 Aug.
14. Lomaira (phentermine hydrochloride) package insert. Newton, PA: KVK-Tech, Inc.; 2016 Sept.
15. Adipex-P (phentermine hydrochloride tablets and capsules) package insert. Sellersville, PA: Teva Pharmaceuticals; 2013 Jan.
16. Suprenza (phentermine hydrochloride) package insert. Cranford, NJ: Akrimax Pharmaceuticals; 2011 Oct.
17. Fastin® (phentermine) package insert. Philadelphia, PA: Beecham Laboratories; 1987 Oct.
18. Phentermine hydrochloride package insert. Newtown, PA: KVK-Tech Inc; 2010 April.
19. Xenical (orlistat) package insert. South San Francisco, CA: Genentech USA, Inc.; 2016 Jun.
20. Alli (orlistat) capsules. Warren, NJ: GSK Consumer Healthcare; 2016 May.
21. Saxenda (liraglutide) injection package insert. Plainsboro, NJ: Novo Nordisk Inc; 2016 Sept.
22. Victoza (liraglutide) package insert. Princeton, NJ: Novo Nordisk Inc; 2016 April.
23. Belviq (lorcaserin hydrochloride) package insert. Zofingen, Switzerland: Arena Pharmaceuticals GmbH; 2012 Jun
24. Belviq XR (lorcaserin hydrochloride) extended-release tablets package insert. Zofingen, Switzerland: Arena Pharmaceuticals GmbH; 2016 Jul.
25. Int J Clin Pract. 2014;68(12):1401-1405. Lorcaserin, Phentermine Topiramate Combination, and Naltrexone Bupropion Combination for Weight Loss: The 15-min Challenge to Sort These Agents Out. http://www.medscape.com/viewarticle/836453
26. Contrave (naltrexone HCl and bupropion HCl) package insert. La Jolla, CA: Orexigen Therapeutics, Inc.; 2014 Sep.
27. Qsymia (phentermine and topiramate extended-release) package insert. Mountain View, CA: Vivus, Inc.; 2014 Sept.
28. Gadde KM, Allison DB, Ryan DH, et al. Effects of low-dose, controlled-release, phentermine plus topiramate combination on weight and associated comorbidities in overweight and obese adults (CONQUER): a randomised, placebo-controlled, phase 3 trial. Lancet. 2011;377:1341-1352. Epub 2011 Apr 8. Erratum in: Lancet. 2011;377:1494.
29. O'Neill PM, Peterson, CA. Weight Loss and Depression in Overweight/Obese Subjects With a History of Depression Receiving Phentermine and Topiramate Extended-Release. Presented at the 166th Annual Meeting of the American Psychiatric Association (APA) San Francisco, CA; 2013 May 20. (unpublished).
30. Allison DB, et al. Controlled-release phentermine/topiramate in severely obese adults: a randomized controlled trial (EQUIP). Obesity (Silver Spring). 2012;20:330-342
31. Addyi (flibanserin tablets) package insert. Raleigh, NC: Sprout Pharmaceuticals, Inc.; 2016 Jun.
32. Dextromethorphan hydrobromide; quinidine sulfate capsule (Nuedexta) package insert. Aliso Viejo, CA: Avanir Pharmaceuticals, Inc.; 2015 Jan.

Alzheimer's Dementia (AD):
1. American Psychiatric Association: Diagnostic and Statistical Manual of Mental Disorders, Fifth Edition. Arlington, VA: American Psychiatric Association, 2013
2. Aricept® (donepezil hydrochloride) package insert. Teaneck, NJ: Eisai Co., Ltd.; 2006 Nov.
3. Aricept (donepezil hydrochloride) package insert. Woodcliff Lake, NJ: Eisai Co., Ltd.; 2015 Jul.
4. Razadyne® (galantamine hydrobromide) package insert. Ortho-McNeil Neurologics, NJ: 2015 Dec.
5. Razadyne, Razadyne ER (galantamine) package insert. Titusville, NJ: Ortho-McNeil Neurologics Inc LP; 2015 Dec.
6. Galantamine hydrobromide oral solution package insert. Roxane Laboratories, Inc.; Columbus, OH: 2015 Feb.
7. Exelon® (rivastigmine tartrate) package insert. East Hanover, NJ: Novartis Pharmaceuticals Corp; 2004 June.
8. Exelon (rivastigmine) capsule and oral solution package insert. East Hanover, NJ: Novartis Pharmaceutical Corporation; 2016 Nov.

9. Cognex® (tacrine hydrochloride) package insert. Roswell, GA: First Horizon Pharmaceutical Corp; 2002 January.
10. American Journal of Health-System Pharmacy January 2005, 62 (1) 35-36
11. Institute for Safe Medication Practices (ISMP). Burns during MRI from patches with metal in the backing. Acute Care ISMP Medication Safety Alert 2016; 21:1-2.
12. Namenda™ (memantine) package insert. St. Louis, MO: Forest Pharmaceuticals; 2006, March.
13. Food and Drug Administration (FDA). NDA Safety Review: NDA 21-487, Memantine, Forest Laboratories, Inc.; August 20, 2003. Retrieved July 12, 2004. Available on the World Wide Web at http://www.fda.gov/ohrms/dockets/ac/03/briefing/3979B1_04_FDA-Safety%20Review.pdf.
14. Namenda (memantine) package insert. St. Louis, MO: Forest Pharmaceuticals; 2014 Aug.
15. Namenda XR (memantine extended-release) package insert. St. Louis, MO: Forest Pharmaceuticals, Inc.; 2014 Sept.
16. Namzaric (memantine and donepezil hydrochloride) extended-release capsules package insert. Parsippany, NJ; Actavis-US: 2016 Jul.
17. Handbook of Psychiatric Drug Therapy" Sixth Edition, by Labbate LA, et al. (Lippincott Williams & Wilkins, Philadelphia, 2010, 256-258)
18. The American Geriatrics Society 2015 Beers Criteria Update Expert Panel. American Geriatrics Society updated Beers Criteria for potentially inappropriate medication use in older adults. J Am Geriatr Soc 2015; 63:2227-46.

Parkinson's Disease (PD)/Restless Legs Syndrome (RLS)/Extrapyramidal Side Effects (EPS):

1. Sinemet® CR (carbidopa-levodopa sustained-release tablets) package insert. Whitehouse Station, NJ; Merck and Co.; 2002 Apr.
2. Sinemet (carbidopa-levodopa) tablets package insert. Whitehouse Station, NJ: Merck & Co., Inc.; 2014 July.
3. Duopa (carbidopa and levodopa) enteral suspension package insert. North Chicago, Il: AbbVie, Inc.; 2016 Sept.
4. Rytary (carbidopa and levodopa) extended-release capsules. Hayward, CA: Impax Pharmaceuticals; 2016 Oct.
5. Stalevo (carbidopa; levodopa; entacapone) package insert. East Hanover, NJ: Novartis Pharmaceuticals Corporation; 2014 July.
6. Lodosyn (carbidopa tablets) package insert. Bridgewater, NJ: Aton Pharma, Inc.; 2014 Feb.
7. APOKYN® (apomorphine hydrochloride, USP) [Prescribing Information]. Louisville, KY: US WorldMeds, LLC; 2014.
8. Parlodel® (bromocriptine) package insert. East Hanover, NJ: Novartis Pharmaceutical Corporation, Inc.; 2003 Mar.
9. Mirapex (pramipexole) package insert. Ridgefield, CT: Boehringer Ingelheim Pharmaceuticals, Inc.; 2016 Jul.
10. Mirapex (pramipexole extended-release) package insert. Ridgefield, CT: Boehringer Ingelheim Pharmaceutical, Inc.; 2016 Jul.
11. Requip (ropinirole hydrochloride) package insert. Research Triangle Park, NC: GlaxoSmithKline; 2016 Sept.
12. Requip XL (ropinirole extended-release tablets) package insert. Research Triangle Park, NC: GlaxoSmithKline; 2014.
13. Neupro® (rotigotine transdermal system) package insert. Mequon, WI: Schwarz Pharma, LLC; 2007 Apr.
14. Neupro (rotigotine hydrochloride) transdermal system. Smyrna, Georgia: UCB Incorporated; 2015 Feb.
15. Cogentin (benztropine) package insert. Lake Forest, IL: Oak Pharmaceuticals, Inc.; 2013 Apr.
16. Cogentin® (benztropine) package insert. Whitehouse Station, NJ: Merck and Co., Inc; 2001 Oct.
17. Benztropine Mesylate Tablets, USP package insert. Spring Valley, NY: Par Pharmaceutical, Inc; 2001 Oct.
18. Diphenhydramine (Benadryl) film-coated tablet (OTC) package insert. Fort Washington, PA: McNeil Consumer Healthcare; 2013 Aug.
19. Benadryl (diphenhydramine) cream package insert. Skillman, NJ: Johnson & Johnson; 2012 Oct.
20. Artane® (trihexyphenidyl) package insert. Pearl River, NY: Lederle Pharmaceutical; 2003 Mar.
21. Comtan® (entacapone) package insert. East Hanover, NJ: Novartis Pharmaceuticals; 2000 March.
22. Tasmar® (tolcapone) package insert. Nutley, NJ: Roche Laboratories Inc.; 2006 Feb.
23. Azilect (rasagiline mesylate) tablets. Kansas City, MO: Teva Neurosciences, Inc.; 2014 May.
24. Eldepryl® (selegiline hydrochloride) package insert. Tampa, FL: Somerset Pharmaceuticals, Inc.; 1998 July.
25. Zelapar (selegiline) orally-disintegrating tablets. Aliso Viejo, CA: Valeant Pharmaceuticals International; 2016 Aug.
26. Symmetrel® (amantadine) package insert. Chadds Ford, PA: Endo Pharmaceuticals; 2007 Feb.
27. Amantadine capsule package insert. High Point, NC: Banner Pharmacaps Inc; 2011 Jun.
28. Amantadine solution package insert. Huntsville, AL: Qualitest Pharmaceuticals; 2011 Jun.
29. Thobois, Stephane, MD, PhD, Clinical Therapeutics/Volume 28, Number 1, 2006. Proposed Dose Equivalence for Rapid Switch Between Dopamine Receptor Agonists in Parkinson's Disease: A Review of the Literature
30. Xadago oral film-coated tablets, safinamide oral film-coated tablets. Zambon (per EMA), Bresso, Italy, 2015.
31. INGREZZA™ (Valbenazine) package insert. San Diego, CA: Neurocrine Biosciences, Inc,; 2017 Apr.
32. Xenazine® (tetrabenazine) package insert. Washington, DC: Prestwick Pharmaceuticals; 2008 May.
33. Xenazine (tetrabenazine) package insert. Deerfield, IL: Lundbeck, Inc.; 2015 Jun.

Made in the USA
Lexington, KY
24 February 2019